Prostate Cancer
and Me

**One Man's Story To Carry
You Through Your Cancer Challenge**

© 2011 Donaldo Herrera Kochackis
Word Weaver Publishing
San Diego, CA

Prostate Cancer and Me
First Edition
Published in California by Word Weaver Publishing
San Diego, CA
www.ProstateCancerAndMeBook.com

Copyright 2011 by Donaldo Herrera Kochackis
All rights reserved

ISBN-13: 978-1475085440

Cover design by Heather Firth and Ken Hailey
Printed in U.S.A. Dove graphic by Christopher Ewing, Dreamstime.com, ©Ackleyroadphotos.

DISCLAIMER: This book is the author's personal story of his experience with prostate cancer, and as such is not intended as a recommendation or endorsement of any specific medical institution, course of therapy, or other approach to preventing or healing cancer or any other disease. The author and publisher assume no responsibility or legal or moral liability for any individual's choice of therapeutic modality, medical treatment, or other course of action.

DEDICATION

To the many doctors and nurses
and the hospital and RMG Clinic staff
for taking such good care of me as I went
through my cancer adventure.
Some of their names have been
changed in the story.

WHAT OTHER READERS HAVE SAID

I felt the author's pain. I enjoyed reading the book, and it opened my eyes. Well written and humorous. Mr. Kochackis is a strong person with a good sense of humor.

–John Hill, Chula Vista, CA

Prostate Cancer and Me *is a quick and easy 'must read' for anyone going through any type of therapy, or anyone involved with a person in any therapy. It took away the uneasy feeling of the unknown and left me feeling the heartfult meaning of 'mind over matter.'*

–Pamela J. Dembowski, San Diego, CA

Thank you for sharing your most private moments to help someone going through similar decisions and procedures. Easy reading, and very informative.

–Gwen Hill, St. Pius X Church, Chula Vista, CA

Prostate Cancer and Me *follows Mr. Kochackis's life from the discovery of prostate cancer through the treatment of it and beyond. If you are facing prostate cancer, this book will help you understand what someone else has been through with the same disease. You do not need to face prostate cancer alone.*

–Mr. Ian Trotter

ACKNOWLEDGEMENTS

Few books are completed without the help and support of others. In my case, I wish to thank Chiwah Carol Slater for turning my notes and stories into a book she shepherded to completion; Jane Ann Schlang for helping me brainstorm ideas for the front cover; Heather Firth for her six original line drawings and proofreading; Matt Slater and Eileen Sprague for proofreading the edited manuscript; and the folks at RJ Communications for their expertise and patient guidance. If I have neglected to mention anyone who was instrumental in the production of this book, please forgive me.

Now, I take this opportunity to express my heartfelt gratitude to all the medical staff from the various departments of Kaiser Hospital and the San Diego Radiation Medical Group who were instrumental in curing my cancer. Thank You!

TABLE OF CONTENTS

A Typical Rectal Bleeding Cycle

Rectal Bleeding and Hospitalization
Life Goes On...

The Day Before the Procedure
Cleaning Out My System
Sigmoidoscopy with APC
The Procedure Begins
My Mad Race to the John
Digestive Disagreement
Questions and Answers

Incredibly Good News!
Am I Cured of Cancer?

Things to Consider
A Final Word
Books You May Find Helpful

About the Author

INTRODUCTION

You are about to enter into a tale of two adversaries squaring off on the battleground of life. Having been present throughout the entire ordeal, I can vouch for the truth of this tale in which I, a mortal human, vow to defeat my opponent, Mr. Prostate Cancer, in his relentless attack on my body.

Mr. Prostate Cancer's objective: to plant his flag of victory over this human being's dead bones. My objective: to prevent this from happening.

If you picked up this book because you want to know what may be in store for you or for loved ones diagnosed with prostate problems, you have come to the right place.

For my part, I vow to portray my experiences in a candid manner, no matter how embarrassing they might be, adding flashes of what I hope is brilliant humor to ease any pain my candor might bring up for you. I shall do my best to inform and entertain you, with an occasional element of suspense and a sprinkling of fantasies and imaginary characters. God forbid that you should walk away thinking of me as just another cancer patient droning on about his remission! (Who, me?)

Let me begin with a confession. (Better to get these things out of the way up front, lest the world accuse me of trying to sweep my dirt under the rug, don't you think?) If you expect to hear me say I stumbled onto the battlefield bedeviled by fear and doubt, as befits a man who has just learned that he has cancer, you're way off base. No, I must say I have almost enjoyed coming face to face with my enemy. I appreciate a new learning experience, and have used my prostate cancer as a tool to increase my knowledge of the killer disease that has fought so hard to shorten my life.

My first bout with cancer came in 1996, when at the age of 65 I was diagnosed with colon cancer. I survived (minus my small intestine) thanks to my good friend, Lady Luck—or maybe it was just plain dumb luck.

Ten years later I found myself facing a second bout with the beast, identified this time as aggressive prostate cancer. Big words... what did they mean? It looked like I was in for some big trouble.

Offered a broad menu of options to choose from, I elected to pursue two proven treatments: external beam radiation to kill the cancer, and hormone therapy to shrink my enlarged prostate. Fully aware of the life-changing side effects I might have to face somewhere down the road, I set survival as my top priority and stepped forward, confident that my doctors (with the help of the Man Upstairs) would lead me to victory.

From the very beginning—from the office examination that identified the enlarged prostate, to the blood tests that uncovered a high PSA reading, to the biopsy that showed for certain that I had cancer, to the scans in search of cancer cells outside my prostate, to the interminable drinking of water and submitting my body to radiation and hormone shots—

throughout the entire process, I have somehow managed to keep my sense of humor intact. I hope you enjoy my silly fantasies and the life-affirming air battle from your seat on my imaginary flying machine.

Throughout the process, I have continued to ask "WHY?" Not "Why me?" (though you'll find that here, too), but "Why this test?" and "Why that treatment?" This kind of questioning enriched my knowledge regarding the treatments I was receiving, knowledge I can now pass on to help you get a grip on what you are up against and some of the weapons you can add to your arsenal as you step up to your challenge.

This little book offers you a front row seat from which to view the unfolding of one man's experience with prostate cancer. My objective is to educate, inspire and enlighten prostate cancer patients, to stimulate their thinking process and provide answers to some of the questions that arise when attempting to select a treatment program that will ensure survival.

It is not my intention to recommend any

specific type of treatment. I made my choices, and others must make theirs. As you move into the story, I will lead you every step of the way as I go through my process in the hope of extending my life. It is my hope that this view into my experience with the therapies I selected will provide you and your loved ones a better understanding of what may lie ahead should you elect to follow a similar path.

I hope you enjoy the book.

1

I HAVE CANCER!
DISCOVERY AND EXPLORATION

MY ENLARGED PROSTATE

On April 8th, 2008, at the age of 75, I went to see Dr. Irma Covarrubias, my esteemed physician, in her office. Dr. Irma had been my guiding light in health matters for a number of years, and I am deeply grateful to her for the mere fact that I am here to write this account.

"Doc, I think you have some idea how active I am, always on the go," I began. It was true. I had a business servicing vending machines, which I later sold to free up my time for writing this book. "For one thing, I am forever carrying cases of soft drinks up flights of stairs to fill my vending machines. Why I came to see you is, I've been noticing lately that I'm so short of breath by the time I get to the top of a staircase that I have to sit down and rest."

"Does this happen at any other time?" she inquired. "Or is it just when you're carrying the soft drinks up the stairs?"

"No. The rest of the time I'm fine, no problem."

Dr. Irma sat down at her computer to go over my health chart. "Hmmm… according to what I'm seeing, your overall health is pretty good. I wonder… are you having any other symptoms? Anything else that's giving you trouble?"

"Well… yes, now that you mention it… I'm uh… I've been having a little trouble passing urine lately. In fact, I was wondering about that, too. Is that normal for a man my age?"

"Depends. Under certain conditions, it could be, yes. Men tend to find that as they age, there can be problems with the prostate gland. I'd say there's a strong possibility that the urinary problem you're describing could be related to your prostate."

She performed a routine examination and informed me that my prostate was enlarged.

So? What now, brown cow? Does that mean I have prostate cancer? My doctor was wondering, too. I could see the gears turning in her mind, devising a plan of action.

"Tests," she muttered. "We'll need a full battery."

"A battery? Can't you just plug me in?"

She didn't laugh at my little joke. "Could be cancerous," she said. "But not to worry. Not all enlarged prostates are cancerous. We're going to need to perform a number of medical procedures to find out about yours, starting with a blood test, which I suggest you get as soon as possible. Talk to the receptionist on your way out, and she'll set that up for you."

Dr. Covarrubias referred my case to the urologist on May 22nd, 2008.

THE BLOOD TEST

As a colon cancer survivor I was already living on borrowed time. Determined to borrow as much as the Guy Upstairs was willing to lend, I took the hint. I made an appointment to get my blood tested the following day.

But though *I* was moving fast, the medical establishment seemed to have all the time in the world. It took them close to three weeks to come up with my test results. *So many lost days! I worried. What if...?*

My fears proved well grounded. My blood tests showed a PSA factor of 10.3, well above normal for a person my age. I had no idea what a PSA factor was, but they told me that a normal reading was 6.5.

Now I'm no scholar, but I did the math. It didn't take a rocket scientist to understand that something was wrong here.

"What does PSA stand for?" I asked.

"Prostate-Specific Antigen," the technician replied.

I looked up the word "antigen" in my dictionary at home, and found: "Usually a protein or carbohydrate substance (as a toxin or enzyme) that when introduced into the body stimulates the production of an antibody." *Whew! All those big words!* What it boiled down to was that yes, it was highly probable there were cancerous cells lurking in my prostate, doing their darnedest to get out.

That wasn't good news. I'd always thought of myself as healthy! But at least I was done with all the tests. Hah! Are you kidding? That was just for starters. The blood test turned out to be just the first of a long line of tests and procedures. Next on the menu would be a biopsy. *Biopsy?* Over and over, I kept hearing that I should get a *biopsy.* Not being a medical student, I had no idea what that was.

I looked it up in my dictionary at home. Webster said, "The removal and examination of tissue, cells or fluids from the living body."

Reading the words "from a living body" took a big load off my mind! Knowing I didn't have to die to undergo a biopsy, I breathed a huge sigh of relief. All this time, I had been confusing the word "biopsy" with a different word, the one people use to refer to a coroner's examination of a dead body to determine the cause of death!

PRE-BIOPSY PROCEDURES

As it turned out, though a biopsy wasn't as serious a matter as I had feared, it wasn't just a matter of showing up at the doctor's office and dropping my pants, either. Throughout this entire cancer adventure, there always seemed to be some stumbling block, something that kept things from moving forward the way they should. In this case, the delay had to do with the blood-thinning medicines. (I had started taking Plavix after my heart attack. What heart attack? Hang on, I'll get to that in due time). It appeared there was some danger the biopsy might cause excess bleeding, and I would need my doctor's permission to be off the Plavix for a week or so prior to the procedure.

I had my first visit with Dr. Jey Chuang, the urologist, on May 28th, at which time he gave me permission to stop taking the blood thinner seven to ten days prior to the biopsy, which was scheduled for October 13th.

Dr. Chuang instructed me to give myself an enema before leaving home the day of the procedure. The day before the biopsy, he gave me six Ciprofloxacin antibiotic tablets and told me to take one that night and a second just before the operation. That's exactly what I did.

THE BIOPSY OPERATION

On October 13th, the morning of the biopsy, I sat down to talk with Dr. Albert Grant. I have to admit I had mixed feelings. This was the day I had been waiting for, but there was a part of me that didn't really want to know the results. *Yeah, right. Good luck with that line of thinking!*

"How many tablets do you have left?" Dr. Grant asked.

"Four. Why?"

"Some patients just can't seem to follow instructions," he told me. "I know that, and that's why I asked that particular question precisely the way I did. Some people would have taken all six tablets when they were instructed to take just two."

"Oh." Why had they given me six in the

first place, if I was only supposed to take two? Maybe I was just relieved to find I had followed instructions okay, and he wasn't scolding me. When I finally did inquire two years later, as I was writing this, nobody seemed to know what the four extra pills were for. Just one of the great mysteries of modern medicine, I guess.

My mind was busy wondering about the procedure I was about to undergo. "Just what are you going to do to me during this operation?" I wanted to know.

"You will lie down on your stomach," he answered, "so I can retrieve the tissue samples."

"And how are you going to retrieve the tissue samples?" I asked, imagining all sorts of scenarios. (I have what you might consider a strange sense of humor, and I sometimes tend to carry a thought to illogical conclusions.) "Are you going to cut a hole in my stomach to get them?" I asked.

He gave me such a long, hard look before answering that I got the feeling he was thinking I might be a candidate for a padded cell. "No," he replied at last with a grim smile and a shake of his head. "I believe the one nearest the prostate — the hole that's already there — should do the trick!"

I was on a roll, and couldn't stop myself. I had to ask just one more question. "Are you going to use magnets?"

"Magnets? What on earth gives you the idea I would use magnets?"

"Well," I said, "I use a magnet on a string to retrieve loose change out of the pond in the park — when no one's looking, of course! I thought maybe that's the way you do it, too?"

Dr. Grant chuckled and shook his head again. "So sorry," he said, "we don't use magnets."

"A knife, then?"

"No, no knife. We use a needle."

"Oh. A needle. That doesn't sound so bad. Any risk involved?"

"Not really. Mind you, there's always the possibility of infection anytime we go into the body, but I don't believe it will be a problem."

"And how many samples are you going to take?"

"About eight," he answered.

"Why so many samples?" It seemed excessive. "Wouldn't one or two be enough to know if I have cancer?"

"Your prostate is divided into two lobes, left and right. You must understand, not all the samples will have cancer in them. I'll need four or five samples from each lobe to arrive at an average so we can determine your Gleason grade."

"What is a Gleason grade?" I asked.

"Your Gleason classification will give the medical staff a reference point for directing your treatment."

"Oh," I said. "I thought you would only take one sample. I guess this is a bigger deal than I thought."

When the going gets tough, my response has always been to look for the irony. Here I was at age 75, thrown into a fight not of my own choosing, a fight for my very life. Who was the fool who coined the term "golden years"? That idiot must still be living in the Iron Age!

The procedure itself proved to be quick and painless, though I could feel the needle plucking out the test samples. As soon as it was over, I got up off the table and went to the restroom to clean myself up.

I was given an information summary form explaining side effects I might experience over the next few days: infection, blood in urine, blood in stool, blood in semen.

"When can I start taking my blood thinner again?" I asked.

"As soon as the bleeding stops," I was told.

In less then an hour the bleeding had stopped, and I went back on my blood thinner medication.

Now, with the biopsy completed and no evidence of any side effects over the next few days, the real waiting game began. Did I have cancer, or not? If I did, I was told, I would have to submit to imaging tests to determine whether the cancer had spread outside the prostate, possibly even into the bones.

On October 20th, my urologist called with the results of my biopsy.

"You know, Donald, you have reached an age at which the body can no longer function the way it did when you were young," he began.

Yeah, well, that's obvious, my mind said. *Whaddaya mean?,* the kid in me piped up. Fortunately, the adult in me knew enough to keep his mouth shut.

"Your biopsy came out positive for both lobes. If you were younger, we would normally perform certain procedures that, unfortunately, are not options for a man of your age.

What?? This is an outrage, my mind said. *Is age discrimination going to keep me from receiving the finest medical treatment my food stamp program can buy?*

The urologist went on explaining the results of the biopsy, but though I listened intently I was having difficulty grasping the significance of his medical terminology. I caught something about my high PSA factor being an early indicator, and something about the left and right lobes—enough to get the gist of his communication. Not once did he say, "You have cancer." That much was understood, assumed, taken for granted.

Ach! Life never gives a sucker an even break. Now I found myself squaring off against a new opponent: aggressive prostate cancer. *What do these big words mean?* All I knew was that it looked like I was in for some big trouble.

Still, the news did not hit me with the force it had the first time I'd learned I had cancer, thirteen years earlier. Dr. Irma's mention of the possibility of prostate cancer had prepared my mind for initiation into the Worldwide Order of Prostate Cancer Victims.

I turned to my wife. "*Te voy a ganar a la tumba,*" I said. ("I'm going to beat you to the grave.")

Hearing myself utter those words spurred something within me. *What? No way am I going to succumb to this new cancer demon! Hell, no!*

14

2

LIVING ON BORROWED TIME

By the time I reached the age of 75, a lot of water had flowed over the dam. In my younger years I experienced a number of events that could have ended my life.

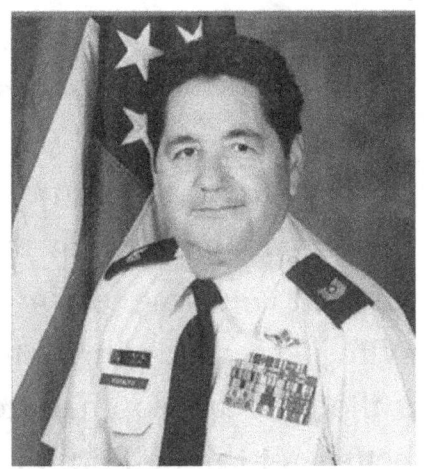

FACE TO FACE WITH A MOUNTAINTOP

One such event came to mind as I thought back to a military airdrop mission that stands out in my memory. We were flying a C 119, a twin-engine flying boxcar. The rear cargo doors had been removed to set up an airdrop configuration, and as loadmaster, one of my duties was to arm the cargo parachute system with the cargo to be dropped. This required that I stand a few inches from the open back end of the cargo floor and reach outside the aircraft to insert the connecting device at a point some 20 inches out—a rather precarious position, to say the least, hanging on for dear life to the netting attached to the load about to be airdropped.

Exactly one minute before we reached the drop zone, a warning would sound to let me know it was time to arm the parachute system. With just seconds remaining before the navigator pulled the airdrop handle, the loadmaster had better get the hell out of the way… or become part of the airdrop! It always seemed to me that time stood still at this point. (This sort of dangerous procedure for arming airdrop loads was later replaced by a slingshot method that eliminated the need to hang on at the end of the aircraft cargo floor.)

This particular night, as we climbed to gain enough altitude to miss some nearby mountains after completing our airdrop, I heard the pilot's voice over the intercom. "Which way do we turn?" he asked, his voice calm and clear. Before the navigator could respond, however, mountains loomed high all around us, blocking our flight path in every direction. "Make up your mind, goddamn it!" the pilot shouted.

Sitting at my duty station near the open space at the rear of the aircraft, ready to jump if the pilot activated the evacuation alarm, I felt the engines being revved up to max power as the commander fought to get this aircraft up and out over the mountaintop.

We passed a glowing red light to the left of the aircraft, probably at the top of some power lines, as we shot up and over the mountain. We came so close to that mountain that I could have reached out and touched it!

We could have all died that night.

I flew for thirty years, and yes, there were other in-flight emergencies. But to this day, this particular night mission stands out as vividly as if it had happened yesterday. I can still hear the panic in the pilot's voice over the intercom, and in my mind's eye I still see the shining red light indicating that we would live to fly another day. Whenever I think back to that night, I remember that I am living on borrowed time.

Some time later, the members of another crew flying in the same general area were not so lucky as we had been. They didn't make it over the mountaintop.

MY UNSUSPECTED PENDING HEART ATTACK

Back in July of 2004, about a week before the heart attack I mentioned earlier, I noticed just a hint of heartburn. If I drank a glass of milk the feeling would go away for a few hours, but then it would return. My wife assured me there was nothing wrong, and I agreed.

Generally, I was feeling all right.

On July 8th I rode the trolley to my security patrol job, as per my usual routine. I was scheduled to instruct a new employee on the procedures involved in making security checks on the buildings we were responsible for. We started at the top of a building and worked our way down. We were about halfway through the procedure when I started feeling strangely uncomfortable. I had never felt this way before.

Explaining to the new employee that I wasn't feeling well, I ended the session and proceeded to my locker to change out of my uniform so I could take the trolley back home.

Good thing I never made it to the trolley! I do not believe I would have made it home. As I was changing my clothes I broke out in cool sweat for no apparent reason. I put my street clothes on and made my way to the front desk. By the time I got there I was in no condition to stand, let alone walk! I collapsed on the floor.

"What's wrong?" a co-worker asked.

"Call me an ambulance!" I requested.

Knowing that I like to kid around a lot, my co-workers didn't believe me. "OK, you're an ambulance!" one joked. "Oh, yeah, we'll call 911!" another teased.

"Call them," I begged, my voice weak.

Once they saw I wasn't kidding, their concern became real and they did as I had asked.

The medical responders arrived and slipped a Nitroquick tablet under my tongue to stabilize me. After a short ambulance ride to the hospital I was placed in the good hands of caring medical personnel. Just in time.

The doctors and the staff took excellent care of me. I was moved to a room full of lights, a very cold room, and pampered with a warm blanket to cover me. IVs, EKGs, TLC. I felt a probe pressing into my heart. *PAIN!* And then it was over, and I was taken back to my hospital room.

Days later, the surgeon came into my room with a group of people. "How are you feeling?" he asked.

Blissfully unaware of the seriousness of my situation, I even felt good enough to crack a joke. "If I was feeling much better, I'd jump up and punch you in the nose!" I replied. *Oops!* I want to apologize for that. Not a nice thing to say to a doctor who had just saved my life.

But I didn't stop there. "Do I still have a heart murmur?" I asked.

Snake Oil Kick-the-Bucket Therapy?

A voice called out, "EKG!"

"Disregard!" another yelled. "Start the blood test!"

"Disregard!" ordered a third. "Bucket!"

Uh-oh. That voice sounded authoritative.

What kind of doctors are running this show, anyway?

The orderly brought out a bucket, and I was given my instructions.

When I heard the command "Kick!," I was to *kick the bucket.*

I did my best to cooperate.

But someone jerked the darn thing out of my reach.

A few more tries.

"STOP!" called the doctor in charge.

"If this patient hasn't kicked the bucket by now, he's going to survive.

Bring out the stent! Installation is now proven cost-effective."

"Yes, you still have a heart murmur," he confirmed.

"Oh… is that why I'm hearing this 'hmm … hmm' coming from my heart?"

This got my doctor's attention! The medical staff standing around my bed couldn't keep from laughing at how my make-believe story of hearing my own heart murmur had fooled the doctor.

Again, I apologize to the doctor. I should have been more respectful. I am extremely grateful for the wonderful care I received at his hands, for all the medical procedures that extended my life. And I am grateful to the UCSD Hospital staff. I was truly pampered.

Once again, I had cheated death. Just another example of why I say I'm living on borrowed time.

Telling you this story now brings to mind five neighbors, all living on the same block, who passed away one by one in a short period of time. The Angel of Death got his hands on my neighbor across the street, and then made his way westward to take two more before crossing over to my side of the street, where he took the last two—including my next-door neighbor. Why not me?

This brings me to the "WHAT IF?" factor in relation to my own heart attack. WHAT IF I had been at home the day of my heart attack? What most people do at home when they're not feeling well is lie down and go to sleep. The hospital medical staff told me that if I had gone to sleep at home I would never have awakened. I would have joined my five neighbors in heaven, or wherever it was they went.

The Powers That Be must have had other plans for me. I'm grateful they arranged for me to be away from home the day of my heart attack. And now, years later, I don't believe they have any intention of letting me slip away as a victim of prostate cancer.

3

PROBING AND SCANNING FOR CANCER OUTSIDE THE PROSTATE

Every time I visited my urologist, I would be asked to provide a urine sample. I would be directed to the room designated for this purpose, and a staff member would come in holding an object with a long handle and a square box attached at the end.

"What's that?" I asked the first time this occurred.

"The sonic equipment we use to check for fluids in the bladder," he told me.

"You sure? Looks to me like a military mine detector—you know, the kind they use to check for explosives."

I was required to lie down on my back while the attendant passed the mine detector over the lower part of my body. When I asked what it had detected, I was always told there was still fluid in my bladder. *Strange!* How could that be? Only a few minutes earlier, I had emptied my bladder to produce a urine sample. What did this mean?

At the first opportunity, I met with the urologist and asked about this.

"What is the significance of having fluid in the bladder so soon after a urine sample?"

"There is a possibility that fluids remaining in the bladder after passing urine could develop into a urinary tract infection," he replied.

"That doesn't sound good. What can we do about it?"

"Well, that depends on you," he replied. "There are things you can do to make sure your bladder is fully emptied. It will be up to you to establish a plan to manage your bladder to assure that it is fully emptied each time you urinate."

I puzzled over that, wondered how in the world I could keep the fluid from accumulating in my bladder. Every time I went to the doctor, the sonic test showed the same result—fluid in the bladder, even after I'd given my all in a urine sample.

"You got some kind of syringe I can use?" I asked. "A turkey baster, maybe?"

He laughed. "No, no syringe, and no turkey baster. You have to do it yourself. The key is to be sure you empty your bladder completely every time."

Well, that may have been a simple thing to say, but I could see that extracting fluid from my bladder that I wasn't even aware was there in the first place was going to take some doing. My thinking process went into overdrive in an attempt to think up a solution to this problem.

I started paying attention to my urinary behavior. I observed that my normal routine was to pass urine, zip up my pants and walk away, only to have to return a short time later to pass more urine. Since I knew something had to change, I would change that. Instead of rushing off after urinating, I began staying two or three minutes after I thought I was done. Sitting there on the toilet seat, my mind relaxed, I found I would experience two or more starts and stops. *Aahhh! There is excess fluid remaining!* And I had discovered how to get it out. Good thing! It might be my protection against a urinary tract infection.

So far, so good! But though that would work at home, it wouldn't be so simple out in the world. Standing longer then usual at a urinal in a public restroom could be embarrassing, I discovered, with men waiting in line for their turn. Absolutely unacceptable.

So... I began using urinals less often. If I had to use a public restroom, I decided it would be better to try my two-to-three-minute drill sitting on the seat in one of the stalls.

THE BONE SCAN

The hunt was on for any cancer cells that might be hiding outside my prostate gland. A nuclear bone scan would be the best way to determine whether there were any, they told me. My doctor scheduled one for November 3rd. If no cancer cells turned up in this scan, it would mean the cancer was still confined to the prostate. If, on the other hand, cancer cells were detected outside the prostate, all bets were off for a quick medical fix.

I didn't like the sound of that. What would I do then? I might as well call home and say, "Honey, you can put this old house up for sale. I won't be using it much longer."

Though I knew I needed this bone scan, I wasn't exactly excited about it. The calendar didn't seem to care about my apprehension, though.

I went into the hospital on the day of the scan, where I was given an injection of 99mTc MOP (short for Medronak) which, I was told, would highlight any areas of bone where active tumors were present. I also received instructions to drink 32 ounces of water over the next three hours.

At the appointed time, a male technician I judged to be about 35 years of age came in with a notepad in his hand. After introducing himself as Mike, he proceeded to fill in some data on a form.

"What are you writing?" I asked, ever the curious one.

"Oh, nothing, just some simple data that's required for the test." He finished writing and approached me. "You're going to need to remove all metal objects and lie down on your back," he informed me. "I'm going to tie your feet together with this strap here. So... if you wouldn't mind lifting them up a bit for me...."

I did, and he slipped the restraining strap under my ankles and fastened it.

"Why are you tying my feet together?" I asked.

"Oh, no worry. It's just to keep them from moving during the test." He pushed the start button. "The scan takes 20 minutes. See you when you're done." He smiled and walked out of the room.

So there I was, tied up like a prisoner, staring down the length of my body at the scanning plates hanging in front of me. Twenty minutes seemed like a long time to lie there immobilized. The table began to move, inching me down toward the scanning plates, causing them to loom larger and larger in front of my face.

I'd never experienced claustrophobia before, but right then it kicked in like gang-busters. Each time I passed under the plates, I had to close my eyes to maintain my sanity. Good thing he had tied my feet! Would they do that when they laid me out in a pine box, six feet under? *At least then*, I reasoned, *pushing up daisies, I'll have plenty of time to get over my claustrophobia.*

Terrorizing though it was, the scan was painless. At last Mike came back in, removed the scanning plates from the apparatus, and took them in to the doctor. Minutes later, he returned with a smile on his face.

"Clean!" he pronounced, handing me the report. "You can go home, Mr. Kochackis!"

Clean! I was jubilant, but I wanted to see for myself. I reached for the report. 'Results of Scan—No metastatic disease detected.' No cancer cells detected in any of my old bones! I breathed a sigh of relief. With my cancer trapped inside the prostate, I knew I had a fighting chance.

THE COMPUTER TOMOGRAPHY SCAN

Next, the doctor had ordered up a computer tomography (CT) scan. I wasn't sure what this scan was for. I figured it was just a backup to the bone scan, to make sure they hadn't missed anything.

I fasted the requisite six hours beforehand and abstained from drinking any fluid for four hours. On November 5th I dutifully presented my ID at the hospital reception desk to a young lady named Helen, an hour and 45 minutes before my scheduled appointment time.

Helen looked to be about 25. Something about the yellow flower in her hair and the way it matched her blouse put me at ease, and when she handed me three 250-milliliter bottles of some kind of drink with a funny short name—'Lafayette Scan C. A. Barium Sulfate Suspension—I took it without complaint.

"Why did they make me come in so early?" I asked.

"Oh, to give you time to finish drinking this 'cool aid,' and to give it time to react."

In spite of the name, it didn't taste bad. In fact, it was sort of sweet. *They say arsenic tastes sweet, too.* I grimaced at the thought. But I drank, because she told me that having the 'cool aid' in my system would give the doctors a better quality readout on the scan. What she *didn't* tell me was that it would either make me constipated or give me diarrhea, and I didn't have the sense to ask her what she meant when she said "react." She must have figured she didn't need to go into detail… after all, I'd find out for myself soon enough.

And I did. *Whoa! I've been blind-sided! Dirty rats!* I jumped up and made a mad dash for the men's room. I was in there awhile. No wonder they'd made me come in so darned early! By the time I came out, I swear I had the cleanest digestive system in San Diego County. When I reported back to Helen to let her know I had drunk all the 'cool aid' and that it had done its dirty work, she directed me to the room where the CT scan apparatus was located.

A smiling woman who introduced herself as Connie assured me that without leaving the slightest scratch this machine would tell my urologist where I stood in my prostate cancer evaluation. Turning to my left, I looked the scanning machine over to see what I was going to be up against.

"What does this machine do?" I asked her.

"It scans your bones using a slicing method, taking pictures of each slice as your body moves in and out of it," she answered.

The "it" that I would be moving in and out of looked sort of like a dark cave. I pictured its walls lined with scimitars. "It's going to slice my bones up?" I shuddered.

"Just visually, Mr. Kochackis," she said with a chuckle. "Don't worry. I assure you, you will come out all in one piece. But you're going to need to drink another cup of the 'cool aid' first," she said, reaching out to hand it to me.

"Am I going to have to make another mad dash to the men's room?"

She must have known what I was referring to, because try as she might, she couldn't keep herself from laughing. "No, I assure you, Mr. Kochackis, that will not happen again."

Reassured, I drank.

Still suffering from residual claustrophobia after my bone scan, I was glad to see that the scanning plates were positioned much higher for the CT scan. There was enough room under them for a big fat pig, and I was a good deal smaller than that. *Oh, good! Those plates won't be passing so close to my face,* I thought.

Connie requested that I lie down on the table, which she offered to help me up onto. She didn't tie my feet together, but she did ask that I try not to move during the scan, which she said would last five to eight minutes. She pushed the 'start' button and walked out of the room.

All alone now, I was pleasantly surprised to find that this time I didn't have any of the unpleasant feelings I'd experienced with the bone scan machine.

Connie returned when the scan was finished and asked whether I felt well enough to stand. She assisted me in getting off the table, and I thanked her for her help.

I was delighted with the results: the CT scan verified that there was no evidence of cancer cells outside the prostate.

4

CONSIDERING MY OPTIONS

THE GLEASON STAGING SYSTEM

Now that I had completed the bone scan and the CT scan, I was ready for my first of two appointments with Marge Forman, R.N., the nurse case manager charged with evaluating my emotional state and my acceptance of the news that I had cancer. I know that cancer brings up a lot of negative feelings in people, but I had none; on the contrary, I was optimistic about my prospects. For me, this was just another day at the office.

Our first appointment was at ten in the morning on November 17th, 2008. Nurse Marge was in her forties, pleasant and well dressed. I asked her questions about my cancer, showing my ignorance, and she enlightened me concerning my cancer classification under the

Gleason Staging System. She began by explaining the "T" factors, and went into detail on my current PSA status. (That's "prostate-specific antigen status," remember?)

"Your cancer was graded using tissue we removed during your biopsy," she said. "The doctor studied your cells under the microscope and graded them from 1 to 10. Low-grade cancers are similar to normal tissue, and high-grade cancers differ from normal tissue in the way the cells are organized and in cell size and shape. The higher the grade, the faster the cancer is likely to be growing. When there is more than one cancer grade in a tumor, which is often the case, we add the two most common grades found in the tumor together to get the Gleason score, which will then be between 2 and 10."

"I see."

"In your case, the most common grade for the right lobe was four, and the second most common was also four. Adding those together, you had an 8 for that lobe. For the left lobe, the most common grade was 4 and the second most common was 5, giving you a score of 9 for that lobe. That's a pretty high number on a 10-point scale. So we have classified your cancer as aggressive, with a T1c status."

Statistically, as I later learned from an article in our local newspaper, *The San Diego Union Tribune*, only one in 35 men age 75 who have prostate cancer actually die of it.

TREATMENT OPTIONS

She handed me an information sheet with the affirmation "I CAN COPE" at the top, along with the American Cancer Society patient referral form and a list of the names and telephone numbers of 53 current patients who were in different stages of cancer treatment as of September 18th, 2008.

"You can contact any of these men," she said. "There's all the information you'll need: names, dates of birth, ethnicity, phone numbers and the best times to reach them, email addresses, the date of their diagnosis of prostate cancer, and their PSA at the time of diagnosis.

Any of them will be happy to talk to you, to share their cancer experiences and offer any support you might need in learning to cope with your prostate cancer."

I thanked Nurse Marge for her offer, but told her I would prefer to stand alone, that I didn't want to begin organizing my life around my cancer. I was determined to live my life in as normal and productive a way as possible, I said, assuring her that I had better things to do than worry about cancer. "I plan to die in an automobile accident," I declared, "at age one hundred."

Though she laughed at that, the expression on her face was incredulous. "But why wouldn't you want the benefit of other people's experience and caring?" she asked.

"Well," I answered, "I feel comfortable standing alone in this. This is my second cancer adventure. I know I'm living on borrowed time, and I'm choosing to face it with a clear mind. I want to put it all down in writing, without the interference of a support group."

When I got home, I put the contact list away for safekeeping and went on living my life the same as I had prior to becoming a member of the prestigious Prostate Cancer Club.

I had decided early on not to discuss my cancer with my family, and I am happy to say they have respected my wish to maintain a code of silence on the subject. While I am not recommending this to others, since every man has to handle his situation in his own way, this choice has allowed me to get my experience down on paper without having to filter it through the lens of family members' perspectives.

HOW AND WHEN A PERSON WILL DEPART THIS EARTH

As I sat there talking with Nurse Marge the question of how long one should live played on my mind. I saw that the whole human race is headed in the same direction: out of here. It's the "how" and "when" that are up for grabs. Maybe my prostate cancer had opened up a window to look into the future as to *how* I might make my earthly departure. If I believed I was going to succumb to cancer, that would still beg the question of *when*. I was optimistic that my upcoming cancer treatments might help me make good on my bet that I'd live to the ripe old age of 100. (*Keep Dreaming!* a voice inside me whispered. *It might be your best defense!*)

It occurred to me that the current condition of the world financial community provided an apt metaphor for living with cancer. I had heard that banks were unable to borrow from each other for lack of confidence in the financial markets. I could only hope that the Bank of Life would have sufficient confidence to extend me extra life credits, that it would allow me to borrow a few more years of life against the collateral of the cancer treatments I was about to receive! If so, I might still win my bet. But that was a *big* 'IF'!

Still, looking back... seven years after my bout with colon cancer, the Bank of Life had doubled my credit by allowing me to survive a heart attack. Truth be told, I'd been living on borrowed time long before that! The Bank of Life had allowed me to live long enough to keep this date with destiny, to join this exclusive club that only patients with prostate cancer are allowed into. What an honor! Who said life wasn't fair?

Maybe my sense of humor had something to do with my continued survival in the face of such great odds. I never pass up an opportunity for a good joke!

Flashback

In the middle of my heart attack,

as I was being wheeled into the operating room in my birthday suit

with a nurse walking alongside holding an IV,

I took advantage of the opportunity to make what could have been the last joke of my life.

"NURSE, NURSE!" I whispered.

"YES?" She looked down at me.

"Please, no peeking!"

"Maybe my joking around at the time of my heart attack offers a clue to why I'm choosing to face my prostate cancer standing alone and living a normal life," I suggested.

"Maybe," Nurse Marge replied. "You do seem to have a good attitude about it."

SELECTING TREATMENT OPTIONS

I asked Nurse Marge whether there were any treatments available for fighting prostate cancer. She affirmed that there were, adding that it was up to the patient facing a cancer crisis to make the all-important decision as to what type of treatment to accept. She rattled off information about five basic treatments to choose from, each with its own set of possible negative side effects.

"In fact," she added, "if you look at the list I gave you, you will see that it includes each patient's choice of primary treatment. Keep in mind that not all patients have the disease, and age and health are important factors in choosing a treatment. Of the 53 patients on the list, six elected "watchful waiting"; five opted for external beam radiation alone; three preferred external beam radiation plus hormone therapy; two chose hormone therapy only; one went for hormone therapy with Lupron; fourteen elected prostatectomy only; three opted for prostatectomy with the male sling; twelve chose laparoscopic prostatectomy; and one decided on prostatectomy with artificial sphincter."

Whew! That was more information

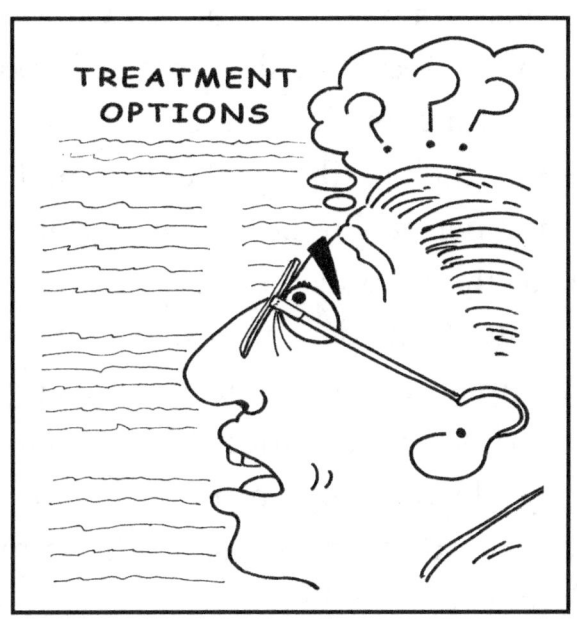

than I was ready to take in.

"Of course, each one of these treatments has its possible side effects," she went on.

"Yeah?"

"Yes. Let me run through that with you, for the top five choices." And she did:

Prostatectomy (removal of the prostate gland): possible blood clots, infection, excess bleeding, difficulty urinating, loss of bladder control, and erectile dysfunction.

Interstitial Brachytherapy (attacking the cancer cells from inside the body by implanting radioactive "seeds" in the prostate): possible erectile dysfunction, incontinence, frequent urination with the possibility of a burning feeling, pain in the perineal region, bleeding or inflammation of the bladder or rectum, and urinary obstruction. Consider also that the "seeds" may be implanted temporarily, releasing a single high dose of radiation, or permanently, releasing decreasing amounts of radiation over a period of months. With permanent seeds you can most likely go home soon after implantation, but you may need to restrict any contact with children and pregnant women for a while. With temporary implantation, you may have to stay in the hospital for a day or more after the first dose, and you may receive one or more doses the next day.

Hormone Therapy: possible hot flashes, breast enlargement, sexual dysfunction, osteoporosis (bone loss), diarrhea, and energy loss.

External Beam Radiation: possible diarrhea, frequent urination, erectile dysfunction, loss of pubic hair, urinary retention and irritation, rectal inflammation with diarrhea, or rectal discomfort and urgent need to pass stool.

Watching and Waiting (with periodic checkups): you never know what might crop up using this method, she said.

"No one can force you to accept a treatment you don't want," she assured me. "It's important to keep an open mind as you listen to the advice of your medical practitioners. They are experienced in treating cancer. But in the end, only you can decide."

After a brief consideration of all the options, I told her I liked the idea of external beam radiation. I didn't have the slightest clue what external beam radiation was all about...except that in my flying days we were trained that to avoid the dangers of uncontrolled radiation we must not walk directly in front of an airplane when its weather antenna was active.

If the radiation from an airplane antenna was that dangerous, I reasoned, a medically controlled radiation beam would give me a good shot now at controlling my cancer.

"Are you sure you understand all of the negative side effects these treatments can cause?" she asked.

"Yes, I believe I do."

"Let me remind you, there is no way to predict exactly what side effects you will experience. No two cancer patents will experience the same negative side effects."

"Yes, I understand." I scratched my head, considering the tremendous quantity of information she had shared with me. "But it is a bit confusing," I confessed. "With all the details bearing on the selection of treatments, and all the unknown negative side effects, I feel like the proverbial little doggie turning in helpless circles — you know, looking first at a tree, then back at his favorite fire hydrant, unable to make up his mind as to where to drain his bladder!"

That got a real laugh out of her. "I suggest you take your time in making your selection," she said when she'd regained her composure. "But don't put it off forever."

No way! I had no intention of allowing any of those demon cancer cells to escape from my prostate and plant their victory flag over my dead body.

"One thing to take into account in selecting your treatment," Nurse Marge went on, "is how it may affect your job. The therapies you're considering may require you to take six or eight weeks off work."

"Oh? Six or eight weeks?"

"You can only be in one place at a time, you know."

Yes, well… I would have to think about that. My job was important to me. Monitoring security cameras and being responsible for locking and unlocking office doors meant I had to walk up and down stairs, which kept me young—no small thing when you've reached the age of 75! I couldn't imagine a better way to stay fit. And the company gave me a regular paycheck, to boot!

(One day, the teller at the bank had told me I looked like I'd been to the beach, my face was so red. "Heck, no!" I had answered. "I'm just embarrassed about cashing this hard-earned paycheck!")

Yes, that job made a big difference in my life. Without the exercise it gave me, I might be a candidate for one of those battery-operated wheelchairs. I saw a senior riding by in one once, and I swear that chair was giving me a hard dirty look, taunting me. *Just wait, Mister!* it mocked. *You're next Ho! Ho! Ho!* How many good years did I have left before I might need one of those? Only the good Lord knew.

Okay, back to reality: how was I going to manage my time so that I could get my cancer treatments and still make it to work on time?

Though work was my prime time concern, it was only one of four considerations that weighed on my mind. One had to do with traveling to and from the clinic: I had visions of being delayed in heavy morning commute traffic and arriving late for my cancer treatments. Another related to the parking situation at the clinic: parking problems are the norm in our society and were to be expected. Finally, I was concerned about my ability to roust myself early in the morning after going to bed late at night. Well, I would have to tackle these problems one at a time, and let the chips fall where they might.

5

Hurry, Doctor! My Cancer Is Trying to Escape!

THE WAITING GAME

I had hoped to get in to see the urologist right away to receive the full results of the bone and CT scans and find out whether he would agree with my choice of treatment program. The earliest appointment I could get, however, was for December 16th.

With time on my hands and no idea how much longer I might live, I started thinking about what I could do in the meantime to keep my mind off my status as a cancer patient. What thoughts would I like to leave to the world? I had an idea for a nationwide network of aqueducts I'd been thinking about for years.

I had been studying ancient history and was fascinated by the foresight it had taken to plan and engineer the Roman aqueducts.

Reading about that had sparked the idea of pumping water from areas of our country burdened with excess water (flooded areas, for example) to higher elevations to create new recreational parks, and then transferring the water via aqueducts to the West, where it was sorely needed. If I wanted any of my self-styled wisdom to survive me, I'd better get busy writing! I dubbed the project 'Aqueduct Westward Ho!' It kept my mind busy during this stressful waiting period.

Though Nurse Marge had counseled me not to rush into any decision, I knew I would opt for the external beam radiation treatment. In anticipation, I began to develop a mental picture of my cancer cells battling to find a way out of my prostate as nature had programmed them to do if left untreated. I was anxious to get started. But on December 11th, my urologist's assistant called to postpone my scheduled appointment to January 21st, 2009.

Was this some sort of sign? I went into a brief panic attack. "Hurry, Doctor Chuang! My cancer cells are trying to escape!" became my battle cry. I pictured them kicking their way through the walls of my prostate. And escape they would, I was certain, just as nature had programmed them to do... if we didn't get this show on the road.

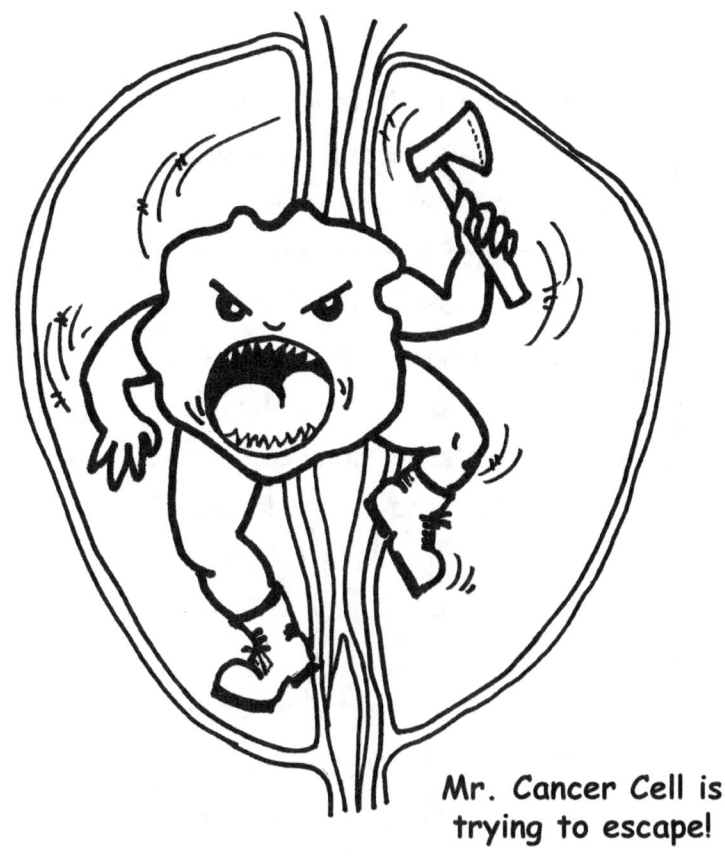

Mr. Cancer Cell is trying to escape!

Why Me, Lord?

I believe the reason I came down
with this prostate cancer is that
I made one big mistake in my life,
when speaking to the good Lord.
I told Him, "Bring It On!"
Oops!
I forgot to add, "Except prostate cancer."
The moral here is that
no matter what we may think,
we are not in control of our destiny.
If we come down with cancer,
we have no choice but to accept it
and go on with our lives.
Now please, don't get the idea
I belong in a padded cell
for thinking this way...
though maybe I do?
Oh, no!
The thought that I'm not in control
of my destiny
is getting a little scary....

GOOD CELLS, BAD CELLS

An idle mind, they say, is the devil's work-shop. Having no desire to let that evil fellow get one-up on me, I decided to put my mind to positive use while waiting for the appointment with my oncologist. I pictured two types of cells sharing the same space in my prostate: the good cells that were my line of defense, and the bad cells — the cancer cells. There wasn't enough space in my prostate for the two to coexist. I imagined those bad cells marching around like ants cooped up in a colony they'd outgrown, fighting to get out and find new food sources in other areas of my body. Those good cells were going to be mighty busy containing them!

Thank God I had the medical treatments on my side. Still, I knew that no magic bullet had ever been discovered for curing cancer. In accepting the available treatments, each cancer patient takes his chances.

I had a full-scale war on my hands — a war of survival.

CHOOSING A RADIOLOGY CLINIC

All the preliminary tests were done, they told me, and it was time to begin the medical treatments that would get rid of the cancer they had found.

I was told I would be receiving the external beam radiation treatments at one of the San Diego Radiological Medical Group (RMG) clinics. I had four locations to choose from: one up the coast, one 25 miles to the east, one 40 miles to the north, and one downtown, just 14 miles up the freeway from my home.

The four considerations I mentioned earlier (missing work, travel conditions, parking, and rousting myself in the mornings) began to fall like dominos on a windy day. First of all, I had the good fortune of being assigned to the clinic located nearest to home, eliminating my concerns about distance and driving in heavy morning traffic.

Then, to get a feel for the parking situation, I made a trial run to my assigned clinic. When I arrived, I found all the parking spaces occupied. It being my nature to look for solutions, I elected to stay and get a better picture of the situation. From my parking place across the street I watched as patients departed and others arrived. I noticed there always seemed to be an available space for new arrivals if they were patient enough to wait a minute or two. So much for the parking concern domino! I've always been a patient man.

As for my concern about missing work, I was handed the solution on a silver platter: I was given the opportunity to select my own appointment times. I opted for morning appointments that would accommodate my three-to-eleven work shift.

Domino Theory Gone Kaput

The last domino fell the hardest...

I was so happy to have all of my basic considerations eliminated that I broke my finger pushing this last domino down the hatch!

(Sorry, I just can't resist a dumb joke...)

Freed of the mental baggage of my four major concerns, I was ready to start my cancer treatments with a clear and relaxed mind.

MEETING WITH THE RADIATION ONCOLOGIST

I went to my January 21st appointment with Dr. Damon Smith of the RMG Clinic. I checked in with the medical assistant, Margaret Delgado, who checked my height and weight, and then with the radiation oncologist, who recommended another blood test.

They scheduled me to come in again on Monday, February 2nd, for a follow-up consultation, and asked me to keep an eye out for a package of documents I would need to fill out and turn in at that appointment.

The documents came, and I filled them out and took them in with me on February 2nd. After looking over the blood test results, Dr. Smith, the oncologist, informed me that he and my primary urologist were in agreement that I should be fighting my war on two battlefronts.

Battlefront number one: the External Beam Radiation Front, where the bad cells would be destroyed. (See? I'd been right in thinking that this was the therapy I needed!) Battlefront number two: the Hormone Therapy Front, where my enlarged prostate would be shrunk back down to size.

Dr. Smith let me know that hormone therapy was no laughing matter, as it presented risks that could be devastating to a person's quality of life. I could end up with hot flashes, breast enlargement, bone loss or diarrhea, and have to drag through each day with little or no energy. None of that sounded good to me! I was at a crossroads, and for a moment I considered rejecting this treatment. But no. I had an aggressive cancer, and a PSA factor of 10.3. It was a no-brainer.

The hormone therapy, Dr. Smith informed me, would begin on February 3rd with a medicine called Casodex to reduce my output of testosterone. I would take one pill a day for two weeks. At the end of the two weeks, I was to stop taking the pills and go to a nurses' clinic and receive a shot. The shots would continue at the rate of one every three months over the next two years. I was also to be placed on another medication, Lupron.

As to the radiation, I was informed that I would be receiving a grand total of 45 radiation treatments.

I signed a consent form to the effect that I understood there could be negative side effects in accepting these treatments. We scheduled my first hormone injection for February 18th and my first radiation treatment for February 19th. They let me choose my own treatment times. I selected 11:20 a.m. for two reasons: I didn't want to have to worry about getting up early in the morning, and lunchtime appointments would create the least interference with my job.

GETTING THE LOWDOWN ON
THIS OLD BUZZARD

Before my first appointment at the RMG clinic was even scheduled I received a call from Melanie at the clinic.

"Are you in a wheelchair?" she asked.

What do they think I am — a little old man riding around in a motorized wheelchair? I laughed. I couldn't resist taking advantage of this easy setup for my odd humor. "Of course not!" I said. "I'm sitting on my bed."

They probably expected that a man of my age would be walking with the aid of a cane. Well, not I! This old buzzard was still walking upright on his own two feet. *For how much longer?* I wondered. *Who knows?*

6

THREE TATTOOS —
I'M A MARKED MAN!

THREE TINY TATTOOS,
CRITICAL REFERENCE POINTS

In preparation for my radiation treatments I was informed that I would be meeting with Charles, the technician, on February 10th to plot the placement of three tiny tattoos, one in the middle of my belly and one on each hip.

"The accuracy of their placement is critical," Melanie told me on the phone, "as they will serve as reference points for your radiation treatments. You'll need to make sure you come in with a full bladder, to help us line the tattoos up properly so that the radiation hits the right target."

"Yes, right. Uh... a full bladder? You want to see me blown up like a balloon? "

She chuckled. "That's right."

"What if I explode?"

Melanie must have heard the doubt in my voice, because she softened her tone. "It's not so bad," she said. "You'll get through it. Don't worry."

That made me feel a little better. It really makes a difference when you feel like the other person is hearing your concerns.

"And there is one more thing I need to let you know," she went on. "Before you come in to have the tattoos marked, you'll need to give yourself an enema at home to clean out any food residue."

Uh-oh.

"So you'll do the enema first, and then before you come in, but after the enema, you will drink 24 ounces of water to guarantee that you arrive with a full bladder."

First I would have to give myself an enema, and then drink 24 ounces of water? All at once? That was three glasses! And then I would have to hold it all the way to the clinic, and all through the marking of the tattoos? I was appre-hensive, to say the least, and I told her so.

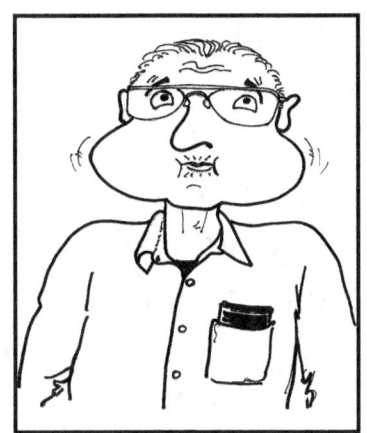

The silence on the other end of the line said it all. I knew I was going to have to comply.

A TEMPEST IN A TEAPOT

The day my tattoos were to be marked I forced myself to stand there and drink exactly 24 ounces of water, exactly one hour before-hand. But it wasn't long before the water start-ed leaving an unpleasant taste in my mouth. I don't have any idea what caused the bad taste; my wife seemed to think the water tasted fine. Maybe my taste buds were rebelling. I grudg-ingly completed the task, trying all the while to keep myself from thinking, *Oh my God, I'm going to have to do this 45 more times!*

But drinking the water turned out to

be the easy part. The hard part? Just as I had thought—refraining from running to the bathroom to relieve myself! Believe me, it was a major struggle of mind over matter. I had already pre-planned the scenario in my mind. I would do everything in my power to delay my visit to the restroom, *no matter how much it hurt,* until after the tattoos were marked.

As for the enema…

People tend to laugh when they hear this word. But believe me, it is not a laughing matter when it is not administered correctly, and they hadn't given me any instructions as to how to do it. I just couldn't seem to master the art of giving myself an enema.

I arrived at the clinic that day with residue and gases still floating around in my stomach. This caused Charles no end of problems. After two attempts to figure out where he should put the marks, he still hadn't been able to make a precise determination. Digging down into his bag of tricks, he took out an item and held it up.

"My secret device for bleeding gases out of the stomach," he declared. He inserted it you-know-where, and immediately I heard a hissing sound.

I heard a voice call out, "Hey, Charley! You got another teapot patient there?"

"Yeah!" he answered. "I just installed my secret device. Whew! This stomach was full of gas."

The "secret device" turned out to be none other than a common soda straw. Ingenious! But it didn't quite do the trick.

Charles took out his tech manual. As he thumbed through the pages I heard him mumble, "Go sit on the stool."

I looked around, but I didn't see a stool.

Charles put down his tech manual and repeated his request. " I have to ask you to go and sit on the stool."

"Where is the stool?" I asked, looking around the room. "I don't see one."

His jaw dropped as he looked at me like I was some kind of idiot. "In the men's restroom!" he hissed.

I sensed he was getting a little frustrated with me. I was probably holding up the next patient in line, all because I'd done such a bad job of giving myself an enema.

After a number of painful minutes sitting on the stool, I was ready for the fourth and final try of the day. If he couldn't do the tattoos this time, he said with a sigh, I would have to come back and try another day.

"And you'd better do a better job on the enema next time," Charles warned.

I climbed back onto the treatment table.

"Here we go, fourth time's a charm," he said. Then, "Bingo! You are a marked man!"

Those three reference points marked me as a ready candidate for my new cancer treatment adventure. We set up another appointment for February 18th, at which time the doctors would check the tattoos to make sure they were in the right locations.

DOUBLE-CHECKING THE TATTOOS

When February 18th rolled around, the doctors did a trial run on the radiation machine (without activating the radiation device) to double-check the placement of the tattoos. Once the final checks were completed, they reminded me that I would have to drink 24 ounces of water one hour before each radiation appointment, and they gave me printed instructions to that effect as well.

I thought about that, about why it had to be an hour before the treatments, and concluded that it must take about an hour for the water to pass from the stomach into the bladder. The bladder needed to be filled like a balloon, I reasoned, to give the external beam radiation machine a direct line of fire as it targeted the prostate from each of several different angles without doing damage to any of the other vital organs.

7

PREPARING FOR BATTLE

HORMONE THERAPY BEGINS

That same day I went to the nurses' clinic for my first hormone injection. Anna, the young lady behind the reception desk, inquired as to whether I had an appointment.

"No, I'm here for my first fix," I deadpanned.

She eyed me strangely, as if wondering whether I thought I was in the rehab clinic. As I approached, my hands shaking, she looked frightened. I was afraid she was going to push the panic button for security backup! But the color returned to her face when I explained that I was there to receive my first Lupron Depot injection.

MY FOLLOW-UP MEETING
WITH THE UROLOGIST

A few days after my first hormone shot, Dr. Chuang commented on how well I was looking.

"How are you feeling?" he asked.

"I couldn't feel better!" I replied.

"Good! You've already received your first hormone shot, and now you will continue receiving injections every 90 days."

It is ingrained in our minds that there is no such thing as a dumb question, but that is probably not the case. I know I have asked some dumb questions in my time. And I was about to ask one now.

"Will I be notified as to when to come in for my next shot?"

He grinned. "This is a long treatment process," he said. "It is impractical to keep track of appointments for every individual patient receiving hormone injections. I highly recommend that you establish your own method of tracking your appointment dates. How about writing them on your wall calendar? That would be a simple solution."

Yes, it would. Why didn't I think of that?

MY FIRST APPOINTMENT AT THE RMG CLINIC

On February 19th, one hour before my first radiation appointment, I dutifully drank the 24 ounces of water, conscious that I was embarking on a test of my endurance that would repeat itself day in and day out until the end of my treatment program. I drove to the RMG clinic and used my check-in card to alert the staff that I had arrived.

In the waiting room the first thing I noticed was a TV set positioned high enough to prevent anyone from blocking anyone else's view. Looking around, I saw three other patients, all talking to each other, sharing their miseries. One of them, a nice-looking lady, held a little dog in her lap. Not wanting to be impolite, I nodded to them. I took a seat in a far corner, closed my eyes, and waited for my name to be called.

As I said earlier, I had elected to stand alone and not join any support group. I didn't want to contaminate my experience with anyone else's stories. After all, I had titled my journal *Prostate Cancer and Me*, and I wanted to keep it that way.

To avoid becoming enmeshed in conversation with other cancer patients and exchanging stories about our respective health problems, I didn't say a word to anyone. Such behavior was out of character for me but I repeated it every time I went to the clinic. I would walk in and see the same three patients but would not say a word to anyone. A simple hand wave was my only way of saying hello, following which I would find a chair in the corner away from everyone else.

If you were one of those patients and thought I was rude or offensive, please consider this a delayed apology. Thank you for understanding!!

MY FIRST "SHOCK TREATMENT"

"Donald Kochackis."

From my seat in the waiting room, I heard my name being called. As I approached the treatment room I saw a group of medical staff standing around and behind the treatment table. They introduced themselves as Henry, Thomas, Albert, Bill, and Jones.

"We're your treatment team," they told me. "And you, of course. You're the most important member of our team. Without you, we'd all be out of a job."

I chuckled, glad to know they considered me a member of the team. I certainly did! I had wanted to come in earlier to meet my teammates and have a look-see at the treatment room, just to get a clear picture in my mind, but I had been informed that state law prohibited such a preview. Well, it was good to meet my team at last. But why were there so many of them? Were we going to have a party? No, the expressions on their faces said we were not. I knew they were all stationed there for some reason… but WHY? That question played on my mind as I walked into the treatment room.

"Drop 'em!" a voice commanded.

I was stunned. This was without a doubt the most embarrassing command I would hear throughout cancer treatment!

"Uh… what? You want me to drop my pants?" I looked around in disbelief at all those pairs of eyes fixed… *on my body!* I cleared my throat to buy time. "You're kidding, right?"

"Drop 'em."

Oh, no. There IS going to be a party, and I'm the guest of dishonor. I was beginning to get the picture. So this was why all those fellows were there!

Before I could say "external beam radiation machine," there I was, standing in my birthday suit in front of a mixed crowd of total strangers.

Had it been up to me, it might have taken forever. But they were on a tight schedule. I gasped as helping hands reached out and unceremoniously pulled down my underwear, exposing the backside of my birthday suit! At least Henry had the courtesy to turn his face away as he held up a large white paper towel to cover my privates.

In My Dreams

Hell! If they'd just played
the right kind of music,
I could have saved them the trouble.

I would have been happy
to jump out of my clothes
before I even got to
the treatment table.

"Sorry, folks,
there is no encore for this act!"

Out of the corner of my eye,
I swear I caught sight of
three judges holding up flash cards:

9! 9! 5!

Hmmm... On a scale of 10?

Not too bad for an old guy!

THE TREATMENT SET-UP

Thomas helped me up onto the treatment table. Good thing! I was none too steady at this point. When they asked me to lie down on my back I complied, clutching that paper towel with all my might, carefully positioning it to cover the area where my underwear should have been. When they tied my feet together I didn't have to ask why. I could see they wanted to keep my body still during the treatment.

But they wanted more.

"Preventing movement is a key factor in guiding the radiation beam to the exact right spots," I heard someone say.

"The three tattoos?" I asked. I knew the answer, but I asked anyway.

"Exactly. We need to stabilize your arms and hands, too. Here, you can slip this rubber ring around your wrists."

"Okay." I reached out for the ring, but I couldn't resist a chance to go for a laugh. "What, no rubber ducky? Can't I have one of those instead?"

"Sorry, not today. You'll have to settle for the rubber ring."

COLD LIQUID GEL AND SONIC TEST

Next, Albert applied a cold liquid gel to my stomach.

"Why the gel?" I asked.

"The gel acts as a barrier between the sonic testing equipment Bill's going to be using and your skin."

"And why do I need a sonic test?"

"To determine the status of your bladder. We have to make sure it's full."

With my body gelled and my bladder full and perfectly lined up for the external beam radiation gun to focus on my three tattoos, I felt really ready to hunt down those cancer cells lurking inside my prostate.

As a matter of fact, I was exhilarated. How many men my age would have rated a 9-9-5 with their pants down?

8

Waging War

THE EXTERNAL BEAM
RADIATION MACHINE

In the treatment room I was introduced to my new ally: the radiation machine.

Looming huge in the middle of the room in front of the flat table I was invited to lie down on, this machine looked like some kind of monster from another planet. Its "business end," the actual weapon designed to kill the cancer cells, was a round radiation device attached to a rotating arm. It would do the dirty work—"dirty" from the point of view of the enemy cancer cells, that is—rotating to stop for a pre-programmed length of time at each of seven different treatment stations to deliver a specific amount of radiation directly at the cancer cells trapped inside the prostate gland.

I was about to receive the first of my forty-five 360-degree cancer treatments.

"I want to understand everything about my treatments," I said. "One question that plagues me is" — and here I confess I did wax a bit dramatic — "Why, why, oh WHY do I have to drink those miserable 24 ounces of water one hour prior to every single treatment?"

"The reason you need to pump your belly full of water every time is so your prostate will line up with the image from the pre-scan," they explained. "The prostate has a tendency to move slightly from day to day. Not a lot, mind you, but enough to require a pre-scan of the prostate, bladder and rectum in order to establish a basic contour image that can serve as a sort of roadmap. We have to make sure the controls line up to the tattoos and aim the radiation exactly where it needs to go every time."

Aah. Understanding that establishing the routine of drinking 24 ounces of water before each treatment would go a long way toward enhancing my chances of survival, I made a vow to myself never to cut corners on it.

"And just which one of you is the man at the controls?" I asked.

"That'll be Jones."

One look at Jones assured me I would be safe with his skilled hands at the controls.

It was time for the treatment to begin. The round radiation device was positioned directly in front of me. As Jones activated the machine from the control room, I heard the sound of it beginning its rotation down my right side. Out of the corner of my eye I saw that it had dipped down to the lower right side of my torso.

The minute the rotation arm stopped, I began counting the seconds to get a better grasp of how much radiation I was receiving. At this first stop I counted off approximately nine seconds before the device started to rotate up my right side. It stopped at my right hip, this time for a count of eighteen seconds. Again it rotated, coming to a stop near the right side of my head for a seven-second count before moving again to stop directly in front of me.

To my surprise, I counted off a twenty-two second pause at this frontal station before it began to move down my left side, stopping to the left of my head for a ten-second count. The next rotation was down to my left hip, for a count of eight seconds. Finally, it moved down to the lower left side of my torso for a six-second count.

Knowing that my counts were but approximate measures of time, I asked just how much RAD (Radiation Absorbed Dose) I would actually receive in each treatment. I was told I would be receiving 180 RAD per treatment.

A 'Twilight Zone' Discovery

That night, I made a weird discovery.
Depending on which lobe of my prostate had received the greatest RAD for the day, the ear on that side of my head would glow in the dark!

It happened every time throughout the course of my treatment. Never once did both ears glow on the same night.

MY IMAGINARY FLYING MACHINE

I lay there looking at the scanner, my thoughts running full speed ahead. *What is this cancer treatment machine all about?* I wondered. I started to imagine its inner workings and the way it would operate to rid my body of cancer.

Searching for metaphors from normal life to help me understand the difference in the number of seconds at each station, I pictured myself as a lawn being watered, with an expert gardener directing more water to the dry spots — the clusters of cancer cells — and adjusting the application as needed to accommodate the inevitable daily changes in the location of those dry spots. The difference being, of course, that this particular bit of gardening was being directed by a computer program.

My mind ran to the years I'd spent flying in military aircraft. I found it natural to imagine the radiation apparatus as my own personal flying machine and assign it the task of gunning down my cancer cells. Once I had created this flying machine in my mind, my next project was to find a way to put it into action. I wanted to develop a program to give you, dear reader, a front row seat in the theater of my war against the attacking cancer cells. I puzzled over how to establish a workable scenario that would give you the vicarious experience of being on the receiving end of these 360-degree treatments.

It wasn't long before a bolt of lighting hit me head-on between my running lights (my eyes). Bingo! The machine stopped at seven points, as described above, to take aim and shoot; I would map out those seven points on a globe (the torso of Yours Truly) divided into seven zones.

THE FIRST GUNNERY STOP

Imagining these flights gave me the impression I was assisting in my own treatment with my imaginary ray gun. The first gunnery stop was in the lower eastern region of the globe, near the South Pole. From there, the attack mechanism gradually worked its way up through the eastern regions toward the North

Pole, and then back down through the western regions until it returned to the South Pole. As for the time duration at each stop, as you recall, I had already pre-counted every second.

MY FIRST FANTASY FLIGHT

Once the technicians had completed all the preparations, the lights were turned off and the technicians left the room. I was ready for my first fantasy flight.

COMBAT MISSIONS

My combat mission: to seek and destroy all enemy cells. The basic rules of engagement: to spot, attack and kill any and all cancer cells found trying to escape. All cancer cells were considered fair game.

I imagined the cancer cells as always on the move, attempting to eat their way out of the prostate from all directions at once. Their mission: to escape and occupy the rest of my body (making my mission harder to carry out) and then go in for the kill.

Who would survive this life-and-death struggle? Only time would tell!

PRE-FLIGHT INSPECTION

As any aviator can tell you, the success of a flight depends in large part on the quality of the pre-flight inspection. In this case, the pre-flight inspection consisted of the checking the panel lights to ensure that they were all in working order. Then, prior to take-off, I would have to read the latest intelligence reports and check firing time durations and the location of the seven critical points.

Once the battle was on, it would be my responsibility to make appropriate adjustments according to the number of exposed cancer cells caught trying to make their escape.

THE GROUND CONTROL TEAM

This combat situation was going to require teamwork with units on the ground. Ground Control would determine the time settings for each attack, with the objective of eliminating as many cancer cells as possible in the shortest amount of time, and send out a drone after each attack to relay real-time intelligence for the purpose of evaluating battle damage.

MY FIRST BATTLE

My mind switched into cyberspace, and I jumped into my flying machine. Within seconds I was flying at low altitude, looking for likely targets. Flying in my assigned racetrack pattern, I received my first alert from Ground Control.

"Warning! Warning! Cancer cells escaping at or near the South Pole! Your firing duration for this target will be nine seconds."

I put my external beam flying machine into a steep dive, guns at the ready. I spotted my target—the cancer cells' leader, down near a hole in the right side of the prostate—and pulled the trigger for a nine-second burst, cutting him down before he could make his escape. Most of the other cancer cells panicked after seeing so many of their kind lying dead or dying on the ground and rushed back to the safety of the prostate. Others ran in confused circles, making them easy targets for my external beam guns.

Ground Control came in on the radio. "Drone Intelligence reports job well done. Climb to 5,000 feet and and stand by for new targets."

Ground Control directed me to fly for ten minutes on a compass heading of 045 degrees. The drone had spotted what looked like a cluster of enemy cells lingering in the region midway between the equator and the South Pole. Another escape attempt?

"Your firing duration for this target will be 18 seconds."

Looking down, I spotted the cluster of cancer cells. I could see an enemy crew working to clear a path by removing the corpses of cancer cells killed in the previous escape attempt.

The enemy lookout spotted me as I began my dive to the target. His warning came too late for about 98 percent of the cancer cells, but another two percent were able to jump back into the protection of the prostate gland. With a large number of enemy cells out in the open, I set my external beam guns to full power and pulled the trigger. What a sight! I smiled at the sight of dead cancer cells flying in all directions, as if blown by the wind. The remaining enemy cells jumped back to the safety of the prostate, where my drone flying cover overhead would keep them at bay.

Eliminating thousands of cancer cells with one shot was a tremendously satisfying experience. Faced with such huge numbers of enemy troops, however, I was unable to complete the job. Furthermore, the cancer cells had found a way to cause a burning feeling, a side effect not to my liking.

Third Attack: I was flying again in my assigned racetrack sector when Ground Control broke the silence with an announcement over the radio.

"*Warning!* Extra-heavy activity between the North Pole and the equator. Your firing duration for this attack will be seven seconds."

The drone's intelligence data suggested the cancer cells were moving in a northwesterly direction. Looking at my maps, I saw that they were advancing into the Mild-to-Moderate Diarrhea Zone, putting me in great danger if my protective equipment were to fail. *Uh-oh!* I had forgotten to bring along a spare sanitary napkin!

I set my sights on their weak spot. With my external beam guns still hot from my last encounter, I pulled the trigger. Diarrhea danger averted. Whew! That was close.

Looking back as I climbed up through the clouds on my way to my assigned air sector and altitude, I had a good view of the damage to the target area. There was little or no collateral damage to the surrounding healthy tissues.

"Congratulations!" Ground Control's triumphant laugh came through loud and clear. "The drone's data shows a clean kill. You can forget about getting diarrhea on this trip. You just shot up their whole house!

Fourth Attack: Flying at 5,000 feet, I stood by for my next assignment. I could hear radio chatter but I couldn't make it out at first because of some enemy jamming device. Tuning the radio to the guard channel, I was finally able to make contact with Ground Control and receive the latest information. The drone had spotted some mysterious enemy activity that turned out to be the cancer cells installing camouflage netting over a wide area near the North Pole to hide their escape exits.

This was a target of major importance, and Ground Control ordered me to test my external beam guns to make sure there would be no malfunction. I was instructed to fire for 22 seconds, concentrating on the smoke markers the drone was dropping on the target. I arrived just in time, destroying the target and thereby preventing the enemy cells from giving me any more of those painful bloating and gas pain side effects.

Once again, I had prevailed. No cancer cells had escaped.

Fifth Attack: As I departed from the previous attack, I heard Ground Control directing me to look to my ten o'clock position, between the North Pole and the western equator region, and report back what I saw. I reported what appeared to be some type of water reflection off the sun. Checking my maps, I could see that it was an area where frequent urination and burning feelings originated.

"You will fire at this target for eight seconds," I was told.

I was in for a big surprise, because as I pulled in for the attack I felt a burning sensation. Concerned, I called Ground Control to ask whether the drone had collected any new data prior to my arrival. I was informed that the cancer cells were putting up a strong defense in this sector, installing mirrors to deflect the external beam gunfire.

"Directly back to your position," came the order.

This time it was not "mission accomplished." It looked like I was in for some unpleasant times—a possible urinary tract infection, courtesy of the enemy cells' smoke and mirror defense.

Sixth Attack: Given my discomforting condition with urinary problems, Ground Control asked whether I wanted to end this mission.

"Hell NO!" I answered. No way was I going to let those cancer cells get the best of me with this urinary problem. I was determined to get my revenge.

"Understood," Ground Control responded. "In that case, you will descend to 2,000 feet and look to your nine o'clock position. The duration of fire for this target will be six seconds. Your objective: to find a healthy bladder somewhere in the west between the equator and the South Pole. The drone reports the enemy is trying to increase your discomfort by blocking the bladder's exit, thereby decreasing urinary flow."

By now I was madder then hell. I didn't want those enemy cells to prevail at my expense. In my anger, I flew in too fast and missed the opportunity to fire at the target—a total waste of time and effort. I was forced to make a go-around.

On the next pass I found the target and fired, but at great cost. In my carelessness I had given the cancer cells a small victory, creating collateral damage—an 80-percent obstruction of my bladder's exit check valve.

Seventh Attack: Ground Control noted a change in my voice when I called in to confirm my orders to climb to 5,000 feet on a new 90-degree compass heading. I reported feeling a little fatigued. "And my urinary problems are not helping," I sighed. "But with six targets completed, this seventh should be a piece of cake!" Strong words I would soon come to regret.

I inquired of Ground Control as to the drone's latest intelligence report, and asked them to repeat my firing sequence for this target.

"The duration of this firing will be six seconds," I was told. "But we have some bad news. The drone was lost when its computer was hit with a virus from the reflecting mirrors at the previous target area. It went down somewhere near the South Pole."

Uh-oh.

"Your mission: attack and destroy all the cancer cells surrounding the Erectile Dysfunction sector. This target is of utmost importance. You will follow a new targeting sequence, starting with cutting off the power source to the cancer cells' mirror defense. You will begin by directing your fire at the equipment sustaining the curtain in front of the mirrors."

I did as ordered and reported that the mirror defense had been neutralized.

Ground Control asked again whether I wanted to abort the mission at this final target, and I held my ground.

"No!" Fatigue or no fatigue, I was going to accomplish my mission and eliminate those deadly cancer cells attacking the sector where the Erectile Dysfunction starts. I was flying down with my hands ready on the trigger....

Then the lights in the room came on. What a disappointment! How would I ever know whether I had accomplished my last mission?

Nonetheless, it had been exciting.

"Oh, boy! What a ride!" I exclaimed on waking.

Having no idea of the process my mind had been engaged in, my team members looked at one another with confusion. I could see it in their faces: *Who is this guy getting up off the table?*

All I can say is, whoever said getting external beam radiation isn't fun has never flown in my external beam flying machine—which I hereby bequeath to future flyers in the hope that you will enjoy the ride as much as I did!

9

FIELD OPERATIONS REPORT

I should explain that although I had been scheduled to receive a treatment each day, there were days we skipped due to machine breakdowns. There were periodic breakdowns all the way through my treatment program.

MY EVALUATION SCHEDULE

I had progress evaluation sessions throughout the duration of the radiation treatments, as follows:

Session 1: Feb. 27, 2009, 7th day of treatment
Session 2: March 2, 2009, 8th day of treatment
Session 3: March 22, 2009, 20th day of treatment
Session 4: March 30, 2009, 24th day of treatment
Session 5: April 10, 2009, 32nd day of treatment
Session 6: April 22, 2009, 41st day of treatment
Session 7: April 28, 2009, 45th day of treatment

At 180 RAD per treatment, I received a total dosage of 8100 RAD (Radiation Absorbed Dose.) That may sound like a lot, but my doctor said that was what it would take to control my cancer.

FIRST PROGRESS EVALUATION SESSION

"You always come in with a full bladder!" the oncology technician observed on February 27th, the day of my seventh treatment. I didn't ask him why he'd said that, but I did wonder, *Doesn't every patient arrive with a full bladder?* I mean… my life was at stake here. I figured that following instructions was the least I could do.

When the session was over, I made my usual quick trip to the restroom. At that point, I had been shot with 1,260 RAD. Out of concern for my well-being over the course of my treatments, the radiation oncologist had scheduled periodic evaluation sessions with the goal of receiving and evaluating my feedback on my experience. The first of these sessions took place immediately after that treatment.

Nancy, the registered nurse on duty, led me into a back office waiting room. It wasn't more than five minutes before Dr. Smith appeared for our evaluation session. Concerned about any side effects I might be experiencing, he asked whether I was tired, and whether I'd had loose or frequent bowel movements, rectal inflammation, hemorrhoids or bleeding. I answered all of those questions in the negative, saying that I had, however, experienced a different problem. I handed him the feedback report I had written up, which I had divided into seven items:

MY FIRST EVALUATION FEEDBACK REPORT

ITEM ONE: I seem to have to pass urine more often now. Not a new item.

ITEM TWO: For a few seconds I feel like I need to go to the bathroom, and then the feeling goes away. I am able to prolong this phase without any problem until I can use the bathroom. Not a new item.

ITEM THREE: I get up a few times at night to use the bathroom. Not a new item.

ITEM FOUR: When I get up in the morning, I feel tremendous pressure in my bladder. It feels awful, as if it is being blocked. When I get to the bathroom, I'm only able to empty my bladder in a weak stream, with about five stops and goes. After that, my bladder returns to normal. This is a new item.

ITEM FIVE: All other feelings, healthwise, seem relatively unchanged.

ITEM SIX: None of my daily activities have changed.

ITEM SEVEN: I drink 24 ounces of water during the hour before my 11:40 appointment. I return home at about 12:55 with my bladder feeling fine.

The session ended on a positive note.

SECOND EVALUATION SESSION

Though my first evaluation was the day of my seventh treatment, I was called in for a second evaluation on March 2nd, 2009, the *eighth* day of my treatment program.

I'm pretty sure it was NOT standard operating procedure to do the second evaluation only one treatment after the first. On the contrary, I believe that the decision to call me in for a second evaluation so soon after my first was triggered by my inability to pass up an opportunity to play the clown. Walking out the door after my treatment the previous day, I'd gone into one of my inane little charades — reeling and stumbling as if about to fall down. The medical staff had jumped to their feet, ready to come to my aid. When they realized I'd been clowning, the expressions on their faces made it clear that this was no joking matter. Believe me, that's one stupid trick I never tried again.

It was at my second evaluation appointment that Dr. Smith gave me a little heads-up. I was going to have to submit my body to another scan, he said, an axial-skeleton DEXA bone density scan.

"But I've already had two scans," I reminded him.

"Yes, I know. But this particular scan is important. I want you to contact radiology and make an appointment."

It is in my nature to strive to understand how things work. On the walk back out to my car, still thinking about the amount of radiation I was receiving, I did the math. I'd been counting the seconds at each stop in my flying machine, and they added up to about 62 seconds per session. If I was receiving 180 RAD per treatment, just how many RAD was I receiving per second at each of the seven stopping points? Dividing 180 by 62 gave me 2.9 RAD per second.

I like to be able to plan, and it felt good to have data I could rely on for pre-planning my flights in my imaginary flying machine. Understanding how many RAD I was receiving per second gave me a better idea of the significance of the difference in the length of the pauses as the machine rotated from station to station around the globe.

THIRD EVALUATION SESSION

I had received 3,600 RAD. My digestive system was working fine but the frequency of urination had increased significantly. Recalling that my visits to the bathroom had been significantly less frequent at the time of my fourteenth treatment, I'd started keeping a written log of the times when strong urges sent me rushing into the bathroom: 12:15 p.m., 12:45 p.m., 1:45 p.m., 2:45 p.m., 3:30 p.m.

The urges seemed to come like clockwork, beginning with a sharp urge that inevitably led to a disappointing dribble of urine.

I developed counter-measures to protect myself against these urges. First and foremost, I learned to mentally override them and avoid rushing to the restroom at the drop of a hat. I found this to be an effective measure. Within a few seconds the urges would be gone and

I would be able to carry on with my normal daily life.

When I felt the need to get out of bed at night I would have to stand at the toilet and wait for the flow to begin, and the stream of urine would be weak. Then there would be a three-minute delay, after which my body would release a second stream of urine.

I informed Dr. Smith of this new side effect of my treatment, letting him know that I believed I had a mixed bag of the incontinence-related side effects described in the medical booklet they'd given me. He listened attentively and seemed to be satisfied with my progress.

THE AXIAL DEXA SCAN

I made the call as Dr. Chuang had instructed and scheduled my axial DEXA scan for the next afternoon.

When I went in for the scan I was given a questionnaire to fill out. Had I had a CT exam in the last seven days? No. Upper GI exam? No. BE exam? No.

Reading the handout, I learned that the purpose of this axial DEXA Scan was to measure my bone mineral density. The measurements, taken at various points on the body, would let my doctors know the strength of my bones.

That date, March 23rd, is one I won't soon forget. I seemed to have reached a turning point, for better or worse, with regard to the radiation treatments. I had become accustomed to forcing myself to hold back the flow of urine. But as I sat in the clinic late that morning, forcing myself to hold back while I waited my turn for treatment, my digestive system became saturated and unbalanced, forcing Mother Nature to fight back. For the first time, I found myself caught between two of Nature's strongest calls — the urge to empty my bladder and the urge to flush out my digestive system!

Our bodies are programmed to experience two phases: first, the eating and drinking phase, and second, the bladder voiding and bowel emptying phase. But I had pre-programmed my subconscious mind to hold back on visiting the bathroom until after completion of the treatment. Now, Nature's warning bells were going off loud and clear, telling me it was time to move into the second phase. *NOW, dummy!* she screamed. *It's time to let go!* But I am a stubborn person, and I would continue to fight Nature. And win! Still, unable to remain seated, I paced the room to prevent the occurrence of a public accident. (I'm not telling you this to recommend that you take such an extreme stand, but only to let you know that drinking all that water is the easy part. It's holding back that's the real test.)

Noting my distress, Nancy, the nurse, suggested I go use the restroom. I had to explain that I couldn't do that because I would lose my full bladder prior to the treatment! Would I be able to hold back, or would I lose it? Nature is one powerful opponent, and who was I to challenge her? I fought hard to maintain control. *No matter what!* Brave words for a cancer patient with one foot near his grave.

But I made it. As soon as the treatment was completed I jumped off the table, got dressed, and rushed into the restroom to take care of my bodily functions. In the end it took calling on divine intervention to save the day, with only seconds to spare. Who says prayer doesn't work? It worked for me that day.

In retrospect, I see that my choice to put off using the restroom for another 40 minutes or so may have created a change in my internal organs, as from that moment forth I noticed that I felt the call less frequently, experiencing less back pressure in the bladder, and when I did urinate it came out in a free-flowing stream. This was a good sign... or was it? I wasn't sure.

By the next day my near-panic condition had disappeared as my bodily functions returned to normal. All of my health issues were pretty much as I'd reported them on February 27th, with no new abnormalities.

REJECTING A UROLOGY APPOINTMENT DATE

About two weeks after the Axial DEXA scan, I received a call from the urology department informing me that I had an appointment with the urologist. When I asked about the appointment date, I was told that it would take place on April 9th.

"What day of the week is that?"

"The 9th falls on a Thursday."

"Could the appointment be changed to a Monday, Tuesday or Wednesday?" I asked. "Because I won't be able to make the appointment on Thursday."

"No, that will not be possible. The department operates on a very tight schedule, Mr. Kochackis."

Being a stubborn old geezer, I wasn't about to give up any days on the job. I finally had my appointment with Dr. Chuang on Monday, May 18th.

FOURTH AND FIFTH EVALUATION SESSIONS

I was glad my fourth evaluation was routine. So far, I had avoided most of the anticipated side effects. I think the thing that had allowed me to dodge the side-effect bullet was my determination to stick like glue to my 24-ounce water rule. From day one, I had been drinking 24 ounces of water one hour before my appointment and making sure not to pass any body fluids until after my treatment.

At my fifth session, the evaluation team wanted to know how many times I got up at night to use the bathroom.

"Oh, two or three times a night, on average, I guess. But last night, I experienced an unforgettable night of bad rest," I told them.

That was an understatement. Every time I'd gotten out of bed and tried to pass urine, that old blocked bladder condition had hit really bad, a strong push-back pressure. I was thinking, *Not now! Please, please don't plug up on me!* And when it finally did start to come out

I had felt a slight burning sensation, like I was forcing the fluids out of my bladder in a really weak stream. And then, a minute or two after it was done, I had started passing fluid again!

Atten-hut! It was as though my entire life was focused around the functioning of my bladder. I recalled the doctor saying that if my bladder didn't drain completely it would increase my chances of getting a urinary tract infection. I hadn't paid much attention the day he said that, but now I saw how it could happen. I had to do something.

That was when I developed my One-Minute Bathroom Delay Rule for draining my bladder. Realizing that not all the fluid would drain out of it at once, I would stand there for a minute after the stream stopped to see whether the flow would recommence.

INCONTINENCE

It's a big word, and it sounds important — all the more so because every time it's used it seems to occur as the first word of the sentence!

And believe me, it is pretty important to anyone experiencing this embarrassing radiation side effect. I was fortunate in that I was never truly incontinent—I always managed to hold it until I could get to the bathroom—but I did have a major challenge with what the medical community calls "types 2 and 3 incontinence," that is, urinary retention and feelings of urgency to urinate and pass stool.

SIXTH EVALUATION SESSION

With 41 treatments completed and only four more to go, I was still waiting to experience some of the "big adverse side effects" I had heard so much about at the water cooler.

OH, YOU'RE STILL HERE!

One day I crossed paths with Nurse Nancy as she was coming out of her office. On her face I saw a look of surprise, as if she thought I didn't belong there.

"Oh! You're still here? I thought you had already completed your treatments," she said.

I laughed. "Didn't you hear? The doctor ordered my prostate gland cooked 'well done'! He wants it sizzling hot when its served!"

Nurse Nancy was in her mid-twenties, a pleasant woman who was always ready to help if I needed an answer to a question about my treatments. I believe she kept my medical chart at her desk, next to the oncologist's office where I went for my evaluation sessions. I would stop at her desk to chat, and one day I told her I was planning to write a book about my cancer treatment experiences. She was most supportive, and I appreciated that.

MY LAST DAY OF EXTERNAL BEAM RADIATION TREATMENT — THE WORST, BY FAR!

I looked forward to April 28th, 2009 with a happy heart. I was about to receive my last cancer treatment!

The day started out on a high note. With 44 treatments completed, I had been bombarded with 7,920 doses of radiation, enough to cook a horse if taken all in one day. The good news was that I had not experienced a single negative side effect beyond my experiences with my bladder. I was still following my routine of drinking that hateful 24 ounces of water one hour before my appointment time. How had I been so lucky? Who could say?

I departed my residence with a smile on my face, thinking this was going to be the last time I would have to force myself to drink 24 ounces of water and fight Nature's strong urges to visit the restroom.

Driving to the clinic, I got the first hint from my body clock that it was time to visit a restroom. *No big deal.* I had experienced these conditions many times in the past, and I ignored it. *I'll get there on time,* I was thinking, *get my last 180 RAD and be on my merry way!*

Why did Murphy's Law have to kick in that day? You know, Anything that can go wrong… will go wrong." By the time I arrived at the clinic the pressure to visit the men's room was nearly overpowering. And as the poet Robert Burns once wrote, "The best laid schemes o' mice an' men gang oft agley." Translation: your plans don't mean a damn if someone's standing in your way.

In this case, "standing in my way" would be an understatement. The clinic staff had made arrangements for a new patient to receive her treatment in my scheduled time frame! *What? Now? No, this can't be!* But it was. I saw her as I entered the waiting room, sitting there waiting to go in next.

Talk about a monkey wrench thrown into the system! My digestive cycle impulses were within a micro-millimeter of a second of creating a public embarrassment, right in the waiting room! I forced myself to keep my eyes turned away from that young lady and did everything I could think of to try to get my mind off my predicament.

At long last the young lady went in for her treatment and I was left alone with the agony of having to hold back. *Just a little longer! Just a little more.* As a last resort I found myself calling for divine intervention.

Finally! It was my turn to go in and receive my last cancer treatment. Every passing second now became an hour of agony. Well aware of how many seconds it took to get through each of the seven treatment stations, I was appalled to note that my predicament was getting worse. The operator had injured his hand, and that handicap was adding extra seconds between stations!

Counting the number of seconds it took the machine to rotate from one station to the next, I had to call on divine intervention yet another time to give me the strength to keep from flinching. The slightest movement on the table risked affecting the critical reference points. They say waterboarding is torture? Try bottomboarding.

At long last my ordeal came to an end and I was allowed to go and discharge my problems in the proper place. I give thanks to the good Lord for helping me overcome this emergency, because without His intervention I could never have made it on my own.

I had completed the last of my external beam radiation treatments. In a few days I would know whether my pre-appointment routine had paid off.

There is probably someone out there who will say, "What a damn fool, going to such extremes! A simple trip to the toilet would have solved his problem." All I can say is, everyone has their own method of survival. I chose this difficult method, and won! Thanks to help from Someone from above, perhaps?

SEVENTH EVALUATION SESSION

I went into the conference room directly after my treatment for my seventh evaluation session. Having received 180 RAD per treatment, for a total of 8,100 RAD, I put my mathematical mind to work. If it takes 2.9 seconds to deliver one RAD, as the doctor had told me, then the amount of radiation I had received came to... 391.5 minutes, which equates to a little over six and a half hours of total radiation.

No wonder they had extended my treatment over 45 days! If I had received that total amount of radiation all in one day, it would have killed a lot more than just my cancer cells. It would have killed ME! Think about it—the radiation is dumb. Stupid. Unintelligent. It couldn't tell the difference between my cancer cells and ME. I would have been left roasting like an over-cooked Thanksgiving turkey!

Extending the treatment over the 45 treatments had reduced my risk of getting hit by the complications and side effects so commonly experienced by radiation patients, and my adherence to the routine of drinking 24 ounces of water before each appointment had paid off as well. Thanks to Lady Luck, I had dodged the worst of the side effect bullets.

FINAL RMG EVALUATION

Those enemy cancer cells had taken a lot of hits! I was anxious to learn who was winning the war.

In May 2009, I received a notice telling

me I had an appointment with Dr. Smith, who had been monitoring my treatments at the RMG Clinic. Sitting in the waiting room, I kept searching my mind to be sure I had a handle on all the questions I needed to ask. I didn't want to be surprised by any health problems that might come up in the future as a result of the radiation treatment.

The doctor entered the room and asked how I was feeling. We conversed a little and he performed a DRE check on my prostate. (That's "Digital Rectal Examination" — performed by hand, not by a computer!)

"Ah, good news!" he said. "Your hormone therapy has done its job. Your prostate has shrunk back to normal size."

"So… does that mean I'm cured of my cancer?"

"No, sorry. That is not something I can determine at this time. The radiation you've received will continue working inside your prostate, and you will have to continue with the hormone therapy for two years. We won't have the final results until February of 2011. At that time, we'll be able to give you an overall evaluation."

Shucks! Well, I did say I was a patient man, didn't I? It looked like I was going to have to be a patient *patient* awhile longer.

Saving Energy...

I was surprised to see the conference room windows draped with blankets.

Dr. Smith entered and switched off the lights.

"Why all this darkness?" I inquired.

"You'll see."

The room began to take on a greenish glow until it was bright as day.

"What's happening?" I asked.

"This is just to forewarn the gas and electric company that your energy consumption may be reduced next month."

I shot him a puzzled look.

"Looks like you've stored up enough energy to light your house for a year! ...

... You see what we can do
with your dead cancer cells?
They turn green after they die.
The brighter they glow,
the more aggressive was your cancer.
My light meter's reading
'High Danger Zone'. "

"And what does that mean —
'High Danger Zone'?"

"Well, let me put it this way:
Had you settled on watchful waiting,
I don't think we'd be holding
this evaluation session today.
The success of your radiation
treatments is evident
in the fact that you survived."

"Snake oil therapy!" I declared.
"Who thought up this
phony energy saving quackery?"

"Shh! Company secret." he said,
raising a finger to his lips.

10

Meeting Murphy's Law Head-On

FOLLOW-UP APPOINTMENT AT 78TH DAY

I had established a friendly acquaintance with some of the radiation oncology staff, who were doing a super job in supervising my treatments. On June 26th I received a call from Melanie at the RMG clinic informing me that it would soon be 60 days since my last treatment and that the radiation oncologist wanted to see me to check how I was feeling. We set an appointment for July 14th, and she informed me that I would need to get a blood test five to seven days before that.

"Oh, dear. Do I have to fast before the test?" I asked.

Melanie giggled. "No," she said. "This will be a non-fasting blood test."

Ahhh! What a relief!

MY BLADDER EXIT
CHECK VALVE ISSUE

When I went in to see the oncologist, I explained about the discomfort I was experiencing with my bladder. I could feel backpressure, like I couldn't empty it completely. "It's like my bladder release check valve is restricting the flow," I told him. "It makes me think of that joke we used to tell as kids — you know, 'Spell PIG backwards and then say the word FUNNY' — as in 'G-I-P funny'."

The doctor stood there staring at me, not saying a word, so I went on. "I know the axiom, 'for every action there's an equal and opposite reaction.' So I'm wondering... could I be heading for a leaky bladder situation somewhere down the road?"

There we sat, the two of us, face to face in dead silence — a silence so overwhelming that a fly landing on the wall sounded to me like it had come in for a crash landing. I finally accepted the doctor's silence as an unspoken indication that my treatments and consultations here at the RMG Clinic had come to an end. I shook the good doctor's hand and left, after thanking him and his staff for the kindness and respectful treatment I had received.

As time progressed, the situation with what I refer to as my "bladder check valve" improved. The feeling of backpressure holding back the fluid went away. However, I did run into the "equal and opposite reaction" I had joked about with the doctor with regard to my bladder exit check valve! Can you believe it? You have to be careful where you let your imagination take you, I guess. Let me explain.

I came up with the analogy of a toy balloon to get a handle on this new bladder problem. Here's how the balloon analogy works: before a balloon is inflated, it just lies there. Once it is inflated and the air is then released, it changes shape and never returns to its original state.

I believe the radiation treatment shrunk my bladder exit valve to such a point that it restricted the flow of body fluid. Now that the treatments are finished, my bladder exit check valve is acting just like a toy balloon. I doubt the valve will ever return to its original shape.

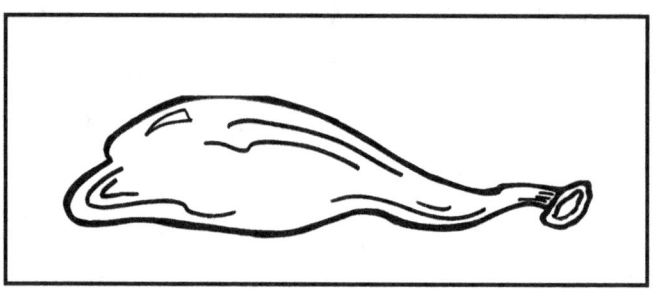

When working correctly, I believe the bladder check valve should open when the volume of fluid in the bladder is ready to be discharged and close when that discharge is completed. But in my case, the bladder drips fluid like a leaky pipe, creating a never ending feeling of needing to pass fluid. The fluid builds up in the urethral canal and telegraphs the brain at the most inconvenient times that I'd better visit the restroom *now... or else!*

The "or else" isn't fun. A good laugh or a movement of the body to reach out for something can trigger a dribble of urine. That means I have to go clean up, or it won't be long before people start talking behind my back. I know, because it happened once when I'd been out running errands with no chance to visit a men's room. An elderly lady in the grocery checkout line turned to look at me, then turned away. A moment later she pointed to me as she whispered to her friend. I couldn't hear the words, but I could read her lips: "He stinks!" I was embarrassed, of course, but I was also grateful for being made aware of the problem.

What to do? The store had an aisle with a variety of costly odor prevention products, but I didn't want to use them. Instead, I developed my own laminated two-piece odor protection system using the trial-and-error method. This system has served me quite well for two and a half years at a cost of only pennies a day.

First, I created a reusable two-part system by putting layers of bathroom tissue between two standard industrial paper towels, which I folded into the desired shape and Scotch-taped in place. Then I created the disposable part of the kit by folding long sections of bathroom tissue to fit the shape of the reusable part. I taped the disposable part on top of the reusable piece, which I use again and again until it too must be replaced. Necessity is the mother of invention!

I still find myself having to deal with the problem of a leaky bladder check valve on a daily basis. This brings up an interesting question: Is there a proven medical procedure to repair a leaky bladder check valve? If not, I'd like to know whether anyone has done stem cell research into rebuilding bladder check valves.

TESTING MY BONE STRENGTH

Airplanes have always fascinated me. After all, I nearly fell out of one.

I took a nasty fall on October 27th, 2009 as I stood out in the street looking up at a plane. I stepped on an uneven section of pavement and fell flat on my face, bloodying my nose and banging up my knees.

"It all happened in the blink of an eye," a relative told me. "You were standing in front of me and then you disappeared! The next thing I saw, you were lying on the ground."

Now you might expect that a fall on concrete would break some of these 77-year-old bones, right? Not a chance. I bounced back up off the ground a few centimeters above the concrete thinking, *Come on, vitamin D, do your job! Save these old bones from breaking!* It worked. This old geezer got up, hurting like hell but with all his bones intact. (Thanks, vitamin D!) I was able to stand and walk into the house under my own power, keeping pressure on the bridge of my nose to stop the bleeding. I may have been hurting but I was not about to baby my pain. I was able to walk it off in a few days.

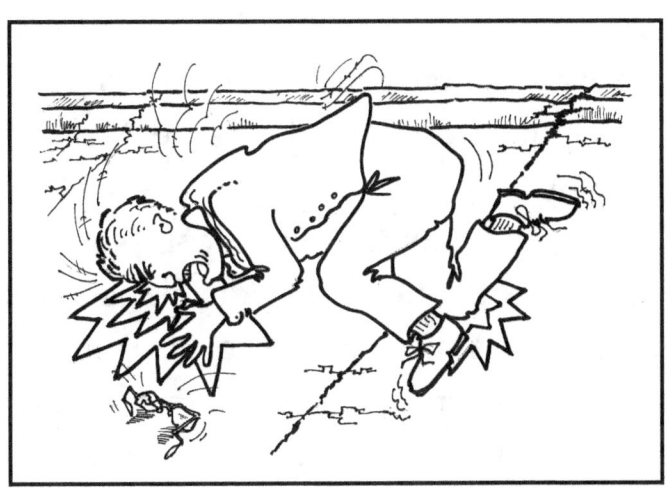

The fact that I didn't break a hip told me I didn't have osteoporosis. I think perhaps the resilience of my bones demonstrates the value of following my doctor's advice and taking my daily 1000 milligrams of calcium and vitamin D. I realized I was doing remarkably well when it came to avoiding the "possible negative side effects" of my treatments.

OOOPS...
LOOKS LIKE I SPOKE TOO SOON!

Remember what I said about Lady Luck keeping me safe from unwanted side effects?

That happy state of mind started to fade on December 1st, 2009, the day I first became aware of a potential problem developing. When I noticed blood on the toilet tissue, I could not believe my eyes.

Over the months since completing my radiation treatments, I had developed what I thought was a simple case of constipation. I had ignored it, accepting it as just another new fact of life after my cancer treatment. The blockage causing this constipation had finally broken loose, giving rise to blood mixed in with the stool in the toilet bowl.

I flashed back to a previous digestive tract bleeding problem my personal doctor had detected. That time, it had signaled the onset of colon cancer. But the bleeding had been covert; I hadn't been aware of it until my doctor had brought it to my attention. Seeing so much blood in the toilet now triggered an acute case of fear of the unknown. I knew I had to see a doctor as soon as possible.

Sure enough, the negative side effects I'd been forewarned about in choosing my cancer treatments had indeed come to pass. Now I had a better understanding of why the doctors had made sure to warn me of all the possible risks and complications ahead of time, including scarring of the rectum and possible bleeding. They hadn't wanted me to be blindsided when and if it happened, and of course they had needed the legal protection. Understanding didn't make the actual occurrence any less upsetting, however.

Things got even worse one day when I looked down to see that the water in the toilet had turned a bright red. And to my horror, I saw that my shorts were soaked in blood. My mind went blank. I just couldn't believe this was happening. But there it was, right in front of my eyes. Up until now, I had experienced a false since of security. I had thought I'd weathered the storm and would not be faced with any of the predicted unpleasant side effects. Could this delayed rectal bleeding be evidence that my prostate was still in the cooking stage, seven months after completing my treatments? Strange, indeed. Unthinkable!

I would need another colonoscopy, my doctor told me. *Groan.*

COLONOSCOPY

My colonoscopy appointment was schedule for 8:30 in the morning, and I was instructed to arrive a half-hour early. The doctors dictated what foods I was allowed to eat beforehand: liquid chicken broth, Jello, Gatorade, no foods marked in red on the handout. So that my digestive tract would be empty for the procedure, I was to stop eating altogether thirty hours before the procedure. They gave me a solution to drink and told me when to stop taking certain medicines. Most important of all, I was to bring a driver for my return trip home.

ISCHEMIA DIAGNOSIS

I must be the luckiest man on earth, because the colonoscopy showed no bleeding in my upper digestive tract. On the downside, however, I was informed that I had an ischemia condition.

"Ischemia? What's that?" I asked.

"The lack of blood supply to an organ or tissue," the doctor said. "It's typical for cases like yours. A small rectal ulcer caused by the constipation that resulted from your cancer treatment blocked the blood flow, and it built up until it broke through."

"So… the bleeding is partly due to my constipation?"

"Yes."

"So how do I get rid of the constipation?"

"You might want to consider using a stool softener."

Following my doctor's advice, I began taking two 100mg tablets of Col-Rate twice a day before meals. The constipation went away, and I hoped the rectal bleeding was a thing of the past too. But the hidden force I kept thinking about finally showed its ugly red face. Large thick gobs of blood reappeared to show me who was in charge of my body... and it wasn't me!

My situation reminded me of the story of a patient who had gone to see his doctor about his stomach aches. When the doctor advised him to have all his bad teeth extracted, saying they were the cause of his stomachaches, the patient took his false teeth out of his mouth and threw them on the table. "WHAT'S WRONG WITH ME NOW, damn it!" he shouted.

Given that the stool softener had eliminated my constipation, I asked the doctor why the bleeding had not gone away. Might being on blood thinning medicines (325mg of aspirin and 75mg of Plavix) due to my heart condition be causing the bleeding to continue? If so, would my doctor give me permission to go off those blood thinning meds long enough to heal the rectal ulcer? I thought about these things, but when I asked my doctor he said there was no relationship between the blood thinners and the rectal bleeding.

The bleeding would come on for intervals of 24 to 36 hours. Between bleeding cycles, I would pass daily stools with no ill feelings of constipation, no sign of blood in the stool. I noted a pattern: I would pass three to four healthy stools within a 45- to 50-minute period, and then, in less then 30 minutes and without any sensation whatsoever, I would find my underclothes soiled in blood mixed with bits of excrement.

Seeing that amount of blood in the toilet water was frightening, but knowing it was only a rectal ulcer caused by my cancer medical treatments, compounded by constipation, made it easier to bear.

TRACKING THE BLEEDING CYCLES

I started keeping track, to see if I could develop some clues to alert me to the onset of a bleeding cycle. I began my tracking on February 5, 2010. Here is the gist of it:

February 5th: Bleeding started at 7:00 p.m. and continued until 11:45 that same night.

February 6th: First bowel movement at 04:15 p.m. with no signs of bleeding, followed with a second bowel movement at 08:16 a.m., also free of blood. 24 hours with no sign of blood! My hopes were running high that bleeding would never start again. *Knock on wood!*

February 7th: First bowel movement at 03:15 am; still no signs of bleeding. Second bowel movement at 07:10 am, again free of blood. Another at 11:00 am, also free of blood. At 2:40 p.m., just short of 96 hours into my tracking, I noted points of blood in the bathroom tissue, reminding me of the water droplets that come before the rain. And my last bowel movement of the day, at 3:30 p.m., showed blood on the bathroom tissue. Still, that was small potatoes... only a few small dots of blood in the stool.

Though no longer jubilant, I was still hopeful.

Then all hell broke loose. At 4:25 p.m. the bleeding started with a vengeance. Horror-struck, I pictured the gate on the "dam" opening to turn loose the blood reserves to flood my clothing, as it had so many times before.

This particular gusher put Old Faithful to shame. Activated by what looked like a big brown bass pushing its way through, the explosion was so huge it filled the toilet bowel with of gobs of black blood.

Bloody Old Faithful

With my rectal bleeding,
I saw myself in competition
with Old Faithful,
the geyser at
Yellowstone National Park.

Which of us would hold out the longest?

ME!

I hoped.

What a disappointment, to have the bleeding return! I had had such high hopes.

What am I going to do now? I wondered. A fresh thought crossed my mind: *Why not end it all? Get on an aircraft and fly up as high as the plane can climb. Then say goodbye to this cruel world. Yes, JUMP!*

Did I forget to mention that I would bring a parachute along, just in case I changed my mind before I hit the ground? (What? Me? Chicken out? Did someone call me "chicken"? I have to admit, they're right!)

Great idea, that jump. But no, I was not going to find such an easy way out. Instead, the price I paid for my cancer-activated rectal bleeding was also its reward: I lived to tell about it.

A TYPICAL RECTAL BLEEDING CYCLE

My rectal bleeding episodes came on unexpected, often at the worst possible times, while I was carrying out my daily duties. When that happened, I would be faced with the necessity of stopping what I was doing to clean up the mess!

You know me well enough by now to realize I have to look for the positive side of any situation. If there was an upside to this unexpected bleeding, it was that the blood had no unpleasant odor. So I didn't have to endure the embarrassment of having people looking at each other saying, "It wasn't me!"

I developed a mental picture of what I thought was happening at the rectal ulcer zone between bleeding cycles. For starters, once the main discharge of blood was completed and the bleeding had stopped, I envisioned blood continuing to flow until it ran into the rectal ulcer, which functioned much like a beaver dam.

That's what I called it — a beaver dam! This dam would begin filling with blood, either slowly until it got so full it ruptured like a toy balloon, or suddenly whenever a big brown "bass" tried to squeeze by. Then all hell would break loose as a bleeding cycle came on with a vengeance.

Fortunately for me, I was always sitting on the toilet when that happened! The blood would explode past the dam, and when I got up

I would see large gobs of black blood filling the toilet bowel.

11

UNEXPECTED SIDE EFFECTS

I received hormone injections as scheduled throughout 2009 and early the following year: May 12th 2009, August 12th 2009, November 12th 2009, and February 12th 2010.

When I went in for my injection on May 12th, 2010, I was in for a big surprise. Linda, the registered nurse on duty, laid the news on me. "Your medical records from your urologist show no record of authorization to receive further hormone injections," she said.

"Uh… there must be some mistake," I replied, taken aback. "The doctor told me I would be on hormone therapy for two years."

"Well…" Linda checked the record again. "I'm sorry, Mr. Kochackis, I have to follow procedures. There is no authorization here for any more hormone shots."

What??! If I hadn't thought my life depended on these shots, I would have walked out of the clinic right then and never gone back. But I couldn't do that. I was not about to give up.

"I don't understand," I said. "If I'm not supposed to be here, then why did Gloria, the nurse who gave me a shot 90 days ago, hand me a note that said to come back today?"

She shook her head. I could see she was as confused as I was. "I'm afraid I don't know," she said.

"Well...can't you at least try to contact one of my two urologists?"

Linda made a few phone calls and finally received the authorization for the injection. There had been some misunderstanding between Dr. Chuang at Kaiser and Dr. Smith at the RMG Clinic, as it turned out. Linda got it resolved and I received the shot, and another one on August 12th.

I was counting the days until my next injection, scheduled for November 12th.

RECTAL BLEEDING AND HOSPITALIZATION

On July 21st, 2010, I went to see my primary doctor to find out why I was still having rectal bleeding. I explained that what generally happened was that I would be feeling sluggish just moving around, but that once I sat down I would feel fine—until I stood up again, at which time a dizzy feeling would come over me. On top of that, breathing cold air often gave me heartburn over the spot where the stent had been implanted in my heart.

"I feel like my stent needs to be moved," I told her, "so I can feel my heartbeat in my ears again."

"I think you should come in for a heart stress exam," she said.

I reported to the hospital on August 16th for the recommended stress test. When I got there, a young nurse by the name of Christine directed me to get out of my street clothes and into the standard hospital garment—you know, the one with the open air space in the back. Then the questions began: Had I remembered to bring a snack? Yes, I had. Did I smoke or drink? No, I didn't.

They drew a few blood samples and left me alone to put my clothes back on. I was directed to a small area within the examining rooms, where I found two other patients eating their lunch. I took out my own snack and sat down in a chair to eat it. I opened a book I had brought with me. Sam, the patient sitting to my right, asked me what I was reading. In the course of our conversation I told him I was writing a book about prostate cancer. Sam was all ears.

"I'm having problems with my prostate too," he said. "Maybe I can learn from your experience."

This first unexpected face-to-face conversation about my story gave me the encouragement I needed to know that I was on the right course with my book, that it could have a major positive impact down the line on the lives of men suffering from prostate problems. Sam and I exchanged phone numbers, and before he departed for his next series of tests he made a point of telling me he would be buying a copy of my book when it came out.

I finished my lunch and was directed to the treadmill room for my next battery of tests. Alina, the nurse on duty there, gave me some last-minute instructions as to what to expect.

"How fast am I going to have to run on that thing?" I asked, feeling a little trepidation as I eyed the treadmill.

"Oh, you won't be using the treadmill, Mr. Kochackis," she told me.

"I won't?"

"No, I'm sorry, you have a heart condition," she explained. She must have detected the note of disappointment in my voice.

Ah, well, the medical staff knows more about these things than I do, I reasoned, and went in for my test. I came out with a good health report.

By the last week in October my sluggishness had increased to the point where normal walking meant slow half-steps. In spite of it all, though, I felt fine. I had grown used to hearing my heartbeat in my ears, so that didn't bother me. Just a normal part of aging, I figured.

But on October 30th, 2010, I had a wake-up call while attending my high school reunion dance. I've always liked dancing, and believe me, I can cut up a rug. That night, however, I was surprised to discover that I felt ready to turn in after the first waltz. It was the same story all evening long—I'd sit down to recuperate between dances, but at the end of every dance I felt exhausted. *This must be more than age,* I thought. I decided to have it checked out.

I waited for the ghosts and goblins of Halloween to come for tricks and treats, and on November 1st I drove to the hospital to ask a few simple questions. Hah! They had a question of their own.

"Are you experiencing chest pains?"

Like a dummy, I said "Yes!"

That simple "yes" set me up for three unwelcome days of confinement to a hospital bed while the medical staff went to work saving my life. I obliged by slipping out of my clothes and into one of those all-too-familiar hospital-issue open-air gowns. In short order they were busy drawing blood, attaching monitoring devices, and inserting IV needles to dose me up with medication. They even wheeled in a portable X-ray machine and took pictures of my ailing chest.

When all the hoopla was complete they left me lying there expecting to be released to go home. But a couple of hours later a doctor came in and approached my bedside. I could see he had something on his mind.

"It's a miracle your heart is still beating, Mr. Kochackis," he began.

"Really?" I gulped. I knew he was right, of course, about my heart still beating. I could feel the pulse in my ears. But... a miracle? What was that about?

"Let me explain. As I'm sure you know, the heart is a muscle, and as such it requires oxygen to function properly." He looked at me as though to make sure I was getting the full impact of his words. "A lack of oxygen passing through it will cause the heart muscle to be overworked, and the body will begin to shut down." He paused as if to let that sink in. "And if there is too little oxygen coming into the heart over an extended period of time, the heart muscle will die."

I sat there absorbing this, feeling a bit unnerved. *What is he trying to tell me?* I wanted to know, no holds barred. "So... are you saying...?"

"I'm saying you're a lucky man, Mr. Kochackis. You were very near to having a heart attack. Your tests show a dangerously low HGB count of 7.0. You need hemoglobin to carry oxygen to your heart, and you have precious little of it."

Oh. Oh dear. I was beginning to get the idea that it would be a while before I'd be sleeping in my own bed again. Oh well... I had never been big on hospital stays, but now, realizing the severity of my condition, I took the opportunity to offer Lady Luck a silent thank you for reminding me that there are no dumb questions. I shudder to think what would have happened had I not come in to ask about my sluggish performance on the dance floor.

"We're going to keep you here for a few days," the doctor went on, "until we can get the blood for a transfusion. Do you happen to know your blood type?"

I did. "A-plus," I said.

He nodded. "Good. We'll be moving you to ER for your transfusion."

The emergency room was on the sixth floor of the west side of the hospital, so I got to do a bit of sightseeing on the journey. Given some time to think about my low red blood cell count as they wheeled me down corridors and in and out of elevators, I realized that the chronic rectal bleeding must have thrown me into an anemic state. Coupled with the blood loss, it was no wonder I was in need of new blood.

In the hospital I was visited by all sorts of medical personnel and received the ultimate in care and service. November 1st passed into November 2nd, though, before they hooked me up to give me the transfusion.

Afterward, alone in my room with the nurse, I asked her whether my heart had stopped. She gave me strange look.

"No... Why do you ask?"

"Because I can't hear it beating in my ears anymore," I replied.

She smiled and nodded. "Don't worry, your heart is still beating," she assured me. "It's just not having to work overtime anymore."

The post-transfusion blood sample showed an HGB count of 9.6, indicating that my heart was now receiving ample flow of oxygen. I really didn't need that to tell me what a difference the new blood had made, though. I was feeling chipper, like I could dance through a whole evening and still have energy for a walk around the block. I had to look at myself in the mirror to assure myself I hadn't physically regressed to age thirty!

I was ready to go home.

WRONG.

"What's the matter, you don't like this lovely home we've fixed up for you?" the doctor chided. "Too bad. I'm afraid you're going to be staying on with us a bit. One more day of observation, just in case that body of yours should turn out not to like all that new blood."

November 2nd was a long day. I know of nothing less entertaining than sitting in a hospital bed feeling like a million dollars while you wait for the hours to pass so you can get out and on with your life. To entertain myself, I began imagining strange scenarios having to do with the origin of all this new blood now coursing through my veins.

I fell asleep pondering that, and my thoughts made their way into a dream in which the hospital staff assigned me the task of finding out exactly where that blood had come from. After a few hours of deep sleep, I heard myself speaking in Chinese.

"Damn!" I shouted. "This blood was made in China!"

LIFE GOES ON...

The delayed rectal bleeding syndrome was still with me, but I had learned to live with it. I recall how shocked I was the first time I saw my underwear red with blood, when I hadn't even been aware I was bleeding. Now, after nearly a year of dealing with this syndrome, I had developed a sort of sixth sense about it. I would get a feeling that let me know when to expect a bleeding cycle to begin. I had no idea when— or whether—these rectal bleeding cycles would ever end. But I accepted the bleeding inconvenience as a small price to pay for the benefit of having my prostate cancer in remission. Thereby extending my life!

I went into the RMG clinic for a follow-up appointment on October 5th, 2010. I had a preliminary conversation with Nancy, the nurse, during which she answered my questions and refreshed my memory as to some of what had gone on behind the scenes during my treatment. When Dr. Smith came in it was like meeting with an old friend. After all, he had been my mentor through the entire course of my treatment. He asked about my overall health and I assured him I was feeling no ill effects other than the continuing rectal bleeding. He suggested hyperbaric oxygen treatment. I'd never heard of it, but I made a note to check into it.

Recalling that I had mentioned to him somewhere along the line that I was keeping a journal, I invited him to read the section of my story in which I imagined turning green — not with envy, but from the glow of all the dead cancer cells after the radiation series. From the expression on his face, I judged that he enjoyed the reading. As we parted ways he paid me the highest compliment I could have expected, saying he wanted to buy my book when I published it.

In February of 2011, I completed the last of my required two years of hormone treatments. I couldn't wait to hear that I had stomped those enemy cells into the ground! I resolved that I would climb to the highest mountaintop to claim victory over my aggressive prostate cancer. Why not? After all, if those cells had won the war they would be dancing on my grave, waving their victory flag over my dead bones!

12

MY SIGMOIDOSCOPY PROCEDURE

Early in 2011 I received a phone message requesting that I report to Intermediate Care Services as a walk-in patient. They told me I wouldn't need an appointment, so I didn't make one. I presented myself at that location on February 15th.

When I arrived there was some confusion as to why I was there. I showed the receptionist, Stella Gonzales, the note from the Gastroenterology Department directing me to come. Stella accepted my explanation, hooked a medical bracelet on my right wrist, and asked me to wait in the reception area until they called my name.

After twenty minutes medical assistant Rosanna Limcolico called my name. I stood up and she directed me to follow her to the examination area, where they issued me standard hospital garb and assigned me a bed.

"I don't need this hospital garb, and I don't need a bed," I informed Rosanna. "I'm only here to have a blood sample taken as directed by the gastroenterology department. If you don't mind, I'll just sit here on the bed in my street clothes and wait for the doctor."

Dr. Thomas Blair arrived after a while and I showed him my notes.

"The last time I was in the hospital," I told him, "there was some question as to whether or not I would need another blood transfusion."

He looked over my notes, called Rosanna in to take a blood sample, and asked me to remain until the blood test results came back.

When the test results came in, they showed that my HGB count had dropped from a high of 9.6 on November 1, 2010, after my blood transfusion, to 8.5.

Concerned about my low hemoglobin level, Dr. Blair ordered a sigmoidoscopy. Another rectal exam! It was scheduled for February 24th, with Dr. Richard Brower at the Department of Internal Medicine, Gastroenterology Division.

As I explained earlier, I had accepted my rectal bleeding as a small price to pay for overcoming my prostate cancer and extending my life. Those little beaver dams in my veins, caused by the radiation treatments, had caused the blood to back up until it would finally burst through and head for the nearest handy exit — my rectum. This passing of blood had been going on for fourteen months by this time.

I had my last bleeding episode on February 20th, 2011, just four days before my scheduled sigmoidoscopy.

The sigmoidoscopy procedure would include argon plasma coagulation to take care of my rectal bleeding. I envisioned it as sort of like jamming a hot soldering iron against the affected veins, thereby stopping the bleeding and allowing the blood to cycle back into my system. I hoped that would put an end to the bleeding. *Good Luck on that point, Charley Brown!*

(As always, my mind was full of imaginings about the unknown. My doctor didn't really come in with a soldering iron!)

THE DAY BEFORE THE PROCEDURE

I was not allowed any solid food during the 24 hours leading up to the sigmoidoscopy procedure, but clear liquids were A-okay, including broth, Gatorade, black coffee or tea, soft drinks, juices such as grape or apple, and all the water I wanted. No alcohol, though! They also let me have Jell-O (as long as it wasn't red), hard candy, chewing gum and popsicles! It should have made me feel like a kid again, but in truth, as a person used to eating three square meals I wasn't a happy camper. Going hungry wasn't my style.

As for my prescription medicines, I was told to keep taking them up to three hours before the procedure—except the Plavix, which I had already stopped taking five days earlier.

CLEANING OUT MY SYSTEM IN PREPA-RATION FOR THE SIGMOIDOSCOPY

They gave me a one-gallon container with some white powder in it so that I could make my own Gavilyte-C- laxative solution. I was to fill it with tap water halfway up to the marked line two days before the procedure, shake it well until all of the white powder was completely dissolved, and then fill the rest of the container with water and add the contents of the attached lemon-flavor powder package.

I placed the container in the refrigerator, because they had told me it would taste better chilled. I wasn't supposed to start drinking the solution until five o'clock the night before the procedure, at which time I would drink one eight-ounce glass every ten minutes until I'd finished it all off. The instructions said not to take longer than three hours. Knowing from experience that this wasn't going to be easy, I used a straw to help me get all the solution into my body within the required time period.

The Gavilyte-C- Solution did a great job

of flushing out my plumbing. Thank God, this was not going to be a repeat performance of the embarrassment I had experienced the day I received my three tattoos!

SIGMOIDOSCOPY WITH ARGON PLASMA COAGULATION (APC)

February 24th, 2011 was my big day!

I arrived at 1:00 for my 1:30 appointment, as instructed. Irene Alieva, one of the receptionists, greeted me at the desk with a pleasant smile. She asked to see my official ID while Jacqueline Willis, the other receptionist, placed the medical ID bracelet on my left wrist. Irene asked me all the standard questions: Had I followed all the pre-appointment instructions? And was there a driver to take me home? I answered both questions in the affirmative.

"And do you have any questions about this procedure?" she inquired.

"Yes!" I replied. "I was told that I would have to be put to sleep. Is that right?"

Irene checked my medical records. "No... No, it looks like you're going to be awake for the procedure, Mr. Kochackis."

She asked me to remain in the reception area until I heard my name called.

After a while, a voice called out my name. "Donald!" It was Amy Vandell, the nurse who was to prepare me for the procedure. She checked my medical bracelet and requested that I follow her to the procedure station where the sigmoidoscopy would take place.

Valene Antonio, the other nurse, was at the station when I arrived, setting up the equipment in anticipation of the doctor's arrival.

"We'll need you to disrobe from your belt down, including your underwear," she said, handing me the standard hospital gown with the opening in the back.

Ah, yes, the opening in the back... for the doctor to be able to perform his duties.

You know me... I'm still the same old jokester I always was. You are in for a silly, off-the-wall story, so hold onto your seat.

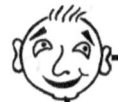

DON'T Let the Sun Shine In!

The nurse asked me to disrobe
from the belt down and
put on the hospital gown,
leaving my backside exposed.

Having completed her duties,
she suggested I relax
and wait for the doctor's arrival.

Suddenly I had this extra-warm feeling
on my open backside,
as if she had turned on a
heat lamp behind me.

How thoughtful!

"Nurse! Nurse!" I called out. "Thank
you for this nice warm heat lamp!
It gives me such a warm feeling."

The nurse came rushing in.

"What's the matter?" she asked.

"I was thanking you for the heat lamp!"

... She laughed so hard
I thought she would split her uniform.

"Ooooh! That's not a heat lamp!"
she managed to say.
"It's the sunshine!"

Now it was my turn to panic!

"Nurse! Nurse!
Quick, pull the shades!"

She did as I asked
and turned to me with a quizzical look
on her face.

"What were you panicking about?"

"Don't you know?" I asked, incredulous.

"Know what?"

"You left me
with my back door open,
letting the sun shine in
on the spot
where the sun never shines!"

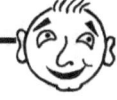

167

THE PROCEDURE BEGINS

When all was ready, Doctor Richard Brower came in.

"So, Donald, are you ready for the procedure?" he asked.

I knew that to him it was a rhetorical question, but to me the question was loaded with portent. While my voice said "Yes," my mind—still holding on to that ugly picture of a hot iron singeing the holes in my leaky veins—screamed "No!"

Mind or no mind, the sigmoidoscopy procedure was on its way. Lying on my left side on the table as Dr. Brower inserted the endoscope, I found myself looking at a monitor on which an image of the area affected by the bleeding sprang to life. For the first time, I was seeing what had been causing my bleeding over the last fourteen months. Studying the image on the monitor, I tried to figure out why the bleeding always came in cycles. I looked to see if there were any extra-large veins that might explain that, but all I saw were small red finger-lines exposing the ugly headwaters of my rectal bleeding. There went my theory about a beaver dam bursting to let the blood through.

"Radiation proctitis," the good doctor said.

"Huh?"

"Medical terminology for 'you have a bleeding rectum.' "

"Oh."

The image on the screen looked to me like a large area of red finger lines mixed with small areas where there were none. The red finger lines began to disappear as he targeted the area with what looked to me like some sort of spraying apparatus. I watched as he directed the spray into one small pocket after another, and little by little those red fingers gave way to white areas appearing on the screen.

"What's that you're spraying?" I asked.

"Argon gas," he said. "This treatment is called APC, short for Argon, Plasma Coagulation. It leaves a thin layer of protective film where the broken veins were."

"And that's why I'm seeing the color change in those areas?"

"You got it." He paused to set something down. "The protective film will disappear, and you'll be left with healthy veins."

I kept watching the argon gas as it eliminated the last of the red finger lines. It gave me hope that my bleeding days were over. *Thank you, Charley Brown!*

Dr. Brower powered the monitor down when the procedure was complete. I was rolled out of the procedure section into the recovery room, where I received my final instructions from Dr. Brower.

"Would you like some pictures to remember this delightful event by?" he asked with a lopsided grin.

"Sure. What have you got?"

"Here." He gave me color copies showing "before" and "after" views of the sigmoidoscopy procedure.

"Well, Doc, I thank you for a job well done!"

"You will have some after-effects," he

warned. "Bloating, passing gas, that sort of thing. Nothing to worry about. It will pass, and after 24 hours or so you should be feeling fine again."

"You can get dressed now," the nurse said with a nod in the direction of my clothing as Dr. Brower walked out of the room.

I did, and returned to the waiting area, where my driver was waiting to take me home.

MY MAD RACE TO THE JOHN

Not long after the sigmoidoscopy procedure, I began to get signs of a war going on in my digestive system. The upper section wanted to pass stool, and the lower section wasn't about to let that happen. Why? I'm not sure. But the upshot of all this was a state of painful constipation.

Time after time I raced to the john, sure that I was ready to pass stool. And time after time, nothing happened.

Under normal conditions Mother Nature provides us with a timely warning when we need to visit the john. But that day, all those warnings were false alarms! Not having eaten any solid food for 30 hours, I had no food in my stomach. And so… no stool. All I did was pass gas.

But of course I did get back to eating once the 24 hours Dr. Brower had spoken of were over. I expected my intestinal tract would return to normal. And indeed it did, but not immediately. My body was going to take its own sweet time.

UPPER AND LOWER DIGESTIVE SYSTEMS IN DISAGREEMENT

After I ate, the upper section of my digestive tract went to work processing the food. After a while, it did what it does so well: it transmitted the message that I needed to pass stool to the lower section.

"I'm ready to send you a load," the upper section called out.

"Whoooaaaa!" the lower section objected. "I'm not ready for that! I just went through a sigmoidoscopy procedure, and my exit gate is barely up to passing excess gas!"

"Sorry, this stool is already on its way!" the upper section responded.

The lower section rebelled by stopping the stool dead in its tracks.

I wasn't in on all this internal conversation, of course. All I knew was that I had to get to the john, and quick! But when I got there, it was the same old story: nothing but gas.

This internal battle between the two sections of my digestive tract went on, over and over, until at last the lower section of my digestive system got so backed up it had no choice but to let the train of stored stool pass through. And while this was going on, I — having no idea whether it was a false alarm or not — would be forced to make a mad dash to the john.

Most of the time I would win the race, but sometimes I would lose.

I continued to experience these false alarms for quite some time. They made me think of the story of the boy who cried "Wolf!" Since I didn't know what to expect, I didn't always take the call seriously.

One time, sure it was another false alarm, I lost the race to the john. That was the first of four such accidents, the biggest of which occurred at 11:45 in the morning on March 1st.

The funny thing was, I had won the race to the john but had passed only a small amount of stool. Thinking I was out of danger, I let my guard down. Then, thinking I was about to pass gas, I was confronted by an explosion so huge that I had to wash all my clothes afterward.

Are you beginning to get the picture of the aftermath of a sigmoidoscopy procedure?

By March 3rd I had made major progress in adjusting to my new alerting system, thus preventing any further accidents. As for the rectal bleeding. Dr. Brower did a hell of a good job. I haven't had any bleeding since February 20th, 2011. Thank you, Dr. Brower!!!!

QUESTIONS AND ANSWERS

At my follow-up appointments with the doctor I had a whole string of questions, most of which he had answers for. Here's the jist of our little Q&A session:

"What is that clear residue I find on the bathroom tissue when a bowel movement refuses to happen?" I asked.

"That clear residue is what the body generates on its own to use as a lubricant for passing stool, if need be."

"So... is the clear residue the plasma you used to stop the veins from bleeding?"

He smiled. "No! The plasma was part of the sigmoidoscopy procedure. It has noting to do with this clear residue. The residue is generated by the body."

"And how long will I continue to see this clear residue on the bathroom tissue without having a bowel movement to go with it?"

"As long as the body needs this lubricant so that it can do what has to be done!"

"Okay, I have a question on a related but different matter. How long before I stop having diarrhea-like stools?"

"That depends on what kind of food

you eat, and how much."

"Okay. Now… What is the meaning of APC in relation to argon? I mean… I know argon is a gas. But what was its function in relation to the sigmoidoscopy procedure?"

"The argon gas is attracted to the red tissue. The argon's function in this procedure was to leave a thin film as it was directed at the injured veins. That film will dissipate with time, leaving the area clean and healed."

"I know the plasma is the liquid portion. But what function did it play in relation to my sigmoidoscopy procedure?"

"The plasma worked in conjunction with the two other aspects of the procedure, the argon and the coagulation. All three of the elements worked together to heal the veins."

"Was the flexible lighted tube — the endoscope — connected to the device you used to spray over the red finger lines?"

"No, no, no. The endoscope is built to stand alone, with telescoping tubing running through the middle of the handle so that the other instruments needed for the procedure can be passed through it."

"What type of special spray apparatus did I see you use to cover the red finger line veins?"

"None at all. I didn't use any other special apparatus. What you witnessed on the screen was the action of the argon gas being attracted to the red tissue. The line carrying the argon gas was passed through the telescoped tubing handle that runs down the middle of the endoscope."

"Okay, I think that's it for my questions about the procedure. Thank you, I appreciate the time you took to answer them. I really like to understand how things work! But I do have a question as to what I can expect. Now that the rectal bleeding has stopped, will my blood HGB count stay at 8.5? Or will it continue to go down?"

"With your blood loss at an end, your HGB Count should remain steady."

"How can I bring my HGB count up?"

"Good question. Start taking iron supplements.

Ferrous sulfate, 325 milligrams daily."

"And when will be a good time to have my blood checked for a new HGB count?"

"You should have blood drawn in about 30 days to get a new reading of your HGB count."

"Why is it that when my HGB was at 7.0, I could hear what sounded like a loud heartbeat reverberating in my ears?"

"That's a question to ask a heart specialist," he said. I got my answer later: At the time of my 7.0 HGB reading, the reduced flow of oxygen passing through my heart had been causing it to work so hard that my heartbeat echoed in my ears.

Deprived of oxygen, the muscle would eventually die. Heart attack! No, I didn't want that.

13

Winning the War

INCREDIBLY GOOD NEWS!

Every prostate cancer patient wants to believe he's been cured. I was no exception.

On September 2nd, 2011, I went in for the first of what I expect to be an ongoing series of post-treatment checkups. My doctor was delighted with the results: my PSA had gone from 10.3 to zero!

"Results like yours bring tears of joy to a doctor's eyes," he said.

His words made my heart sing. I had never heard a doctor say anything like that.

When I set out to write this boook, I had no way to know whether I would emerge victorious over the enemy that had its sights set on taking me down to an early grave.

AM I CURED OF CANCER?

My battle with cancer has brought up a lot of questions for me. A few days after my sigmoidoscopy procedure (the last major treatment I received), noting that my doctor had never used the word "cured," I went to the library to do some research.

There I found *The American Cancer Society's Complete Guide to Prostate Cancer.*

Opening the book to see what the authorities had to say about a cure, I found the following disclaimer: "The information in this book is not intended as medical advice and should not be relied upon as a substitute for talking with your doctor."

Well said. With this disclaimer in mind, I feel comfortable at this point about injecting some of my findings in answer to my question: Having completed my treatments, can I consider myself cured of cancer?

Looking through the Table of Contents, my eyes stopped at the title of chapter 29: "Recurrence." Reading that chapter, I learned that the real answer to that all-important question is neither "Yes" nor "No," but something more like "Time will tell." Why? Because there is a possibility of recurrence within five to fifteen or more years after completion of treatment.

What causes recurrence? It seems that residual cancer cells may survive and lurk hidden even in the best of cases. If left undetected, these bad guys can grow and spread to the rest of the body. The key word here is MONITORING!

So... though I like to think of myself as cured, it may be more accurate to think of cancer as a chronic disease that needs to be monitored over the remainder of your life.

What kind of monitoring should you do? My doctor told me that regular blood tests would be the main indicator that the prostate remains cancer-free. I am to go in for a PSA check once every four months, and twice a year for a DRE (digital rectal exam). As long as my prostate-specific antigen (PSA) levels remain at a safe level (6.5) for my age group, my doctor says I have no worries.

Hence my visit to the doctor on September 2nd. Halleleujah! I am so very grateful.

And yes, I will continue to go in for those regular checkups. At this point in time, I am the winner of this war! And I intend to keep it that way.

THE END

AFTERWORD

THINGS TO CONSIDER

Facing my own bout with cancer, I refused to be overtaken by anxiety. I am a stubborn old coot, and I figured cancer was just another of the many "rewards" of getting old.

I never asked the Good Lord, "Why me?" The only time I did get a little anxious and apprehensive was when my appointment with the doctor had to be delayed.

Having no desire to worry my family over this matter, I made the decision to face this medical problem alone. I never talked with my wife and family about my cancer.

Prayer and a sense of humor have sustained me through the many challenges of my life, and I saw no need to make this life-threatening illness an exception to that. I found the emotional support I needed through the power of prayer for strength. That decision was right for me. A similar decision may or may not be right for you. Your choices may turn out to be vastly different from mine. Please consider your own emotional health and where you will find the support you need to face your situation.

If you do invite your loved ones to get involved in helping you choose between different treatment options, in considering their side effects and supporting you through your treatment, you may be well advised to seek outside assistance as well.

There are established professional groups that will be most happy to assist you through your process, including offering insight into how to help your friends and family deal with their fear for your life.

If you are employed, you may need to consider the effects your illness could have on your work, including how you will handle conflicts between work time and doctor appointments should the need arise. These professional groups can also help you figure out the best way to approach such issues.

Take heart! There is help out there for the asking. And it is perfectly acceptable to ask.

A FINAL WORD

My journey through my cancer treatment adventure was not as easy as you might gather from reading my story. There were times when everything seemed to go wrong. Only a well-seasoned sense of humor saved me from losing my mind! (Much as the doctors, with a little help from my old friend Lady Luck, saved me—again—from losing my life.)

I hope that reading this book has helped you to feel better about listening to your doctor's advice—and then daring to make your own decision as to what kind of care you wish to receive.

Warning: We're talking about your life here. After you choose your treatment, it is up to you to make sure your doctors understand what you're going through. During the treatment process, you must take an active role in your own healing by insisting on real answers to your questions and a pro-active approach by your doctors to handling any negative side effects that may arise. If you don't understand what's happening to your body, it's altogether too easy to justify letting things slide, thinking they must know something they're not telling you. They may. Or they may not.

I am not sure my doctors understood how bad my rectal bleeding problem was. Had I known then what I know now, I would have insisted they do something to stop it when it first occurred. Instead, I waited a year and a half, unaware of the danger to my heart.

If you're Internet savvy, you can check out your symptoms online. If you experience side effects that seem out of the ordinary or excessive, don't wait. Keep insisting until your doctors take active steps to reverse them.

Beyond that, what can you do to increase your chances of winning your war? Calling on my own experience, I credit three non-medical things I did for contributing to my success.

First, I relied on The Guy Upstairs from the get-go. And he didn't disappoint me.

Second, I give my wacky sense of humor a lot of credit for my ZERO (!!) PSA score.

And third, imagining myself battling the army of cancer cells in my flying machine may have had a positive effect. And what about my 9-9-5 rating? That was pretty empowering, too! (If you're a Doubting Thomas, go online and check out the growing body of research confirming the power of mind over matter.)

So remember: prayer, laughter and imagination really are good medicine. You have the right to ask for help from Above. And when misunderstandings arise, as they inevitably will, I encourage you to put yourself in the other person's shoes and crack a little joke, for we do not live in a perfect world. Finally, instead of worrying, why not set up your own cancer-fighting machine?

You never know — these might turn out to be the secret weapons that make the difference between a long life and an early grave!

BOOKS YOU MAY FIND HELPFUL

As I have stated many times in this story, I elected to stand alone in my struggles with prostate cancer. Only after my cancer was in remission and I had competed writing this book did I go looking for information about prostate cancer. I found a lot of medical information but not a single personal story describing what it feels like to go through the actual treatment procedures.

Here are some medical books you may want to consult:

Dr. Katz's Guide to Prostate Health: From Conventional to Holistic Therapies; Aaron E. Katz, M.D.; Freedom Press; 2005; ISBN: 1-893910-37-7.

Prostate Cancer for Dummies; Dr. Paul H. Lange and Christine Adamec; Wiley Pub. ISBN: 0-7645-1974-3.

The Prostate: everything you need to know; Yosh Taguchi, M.D., and Adrian Waller; Firefly Books; 2001; ISBN: 1-55209-553-3.

Dr. Peter Scardino's Prostate Book: The Complete Guide to Overcoming Prostate Cancer; Peter Scardino and Judith Kalman; DIANE Publishing Co.; 2010; ISBN: 1-58333-393-2.

The Prostate Health Program: A Guide to Preventing and Controlling Prostate Cancer; Daniel W. Nixon, M.D. and Max Gomez, Ph.D.; Simon and Schuster; 2007; ISBN: 07432-5432-5.

Mayo Clinic on Prostate Health; David M. Barrett; Mayo Clinic; 2000; ISBN: 1-893005-03-8.

American Cancer Society's Complete Guide to Prostate Cancer; David G. Bostwick; American Cancer Society; 2005; ISBN: 0-944235-54-9.

Invasion of the Prostate Snatchers: No More Unnecessary Biopsies, Radical Treatment or Loss of Sexual Potency; Ralph Blum and Mark Scholz, M.D.; 2010; ISBN: 1-59051-342-8.

ABOUT THE AUTHOR

Donaldo Herrera Kochackis has spent much of his life serving his country. On April 19th, 1949, he joined the U.S. National Guard in California. From 1952 to 1956 he was on active duty 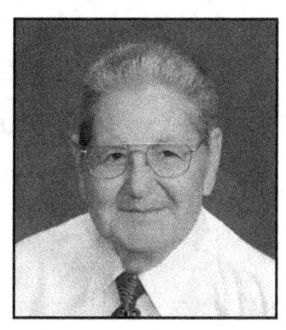 in the U.S. Air Force in the arctic region and in Europe. After that, he served in the Air Force Reserves until 1990, flying cargo planes (C119, C124, and C141). From 1966 to 1973 he flew support missions to Vietnam. In 1975 he participated in the Saigon evacuation, and in 1987 he was assigned to bringing back MIAs from Hanoi. His last wartime missions were carried out in Operation Desert Storm.

Donaldo owned a vending machine business for many years. His creative mind came up with two types of security devices to protect vending machines, and he holds patents on both of them (patent nos. 4566296 and 4350032). He retired and sold the business to write this story.

Donaldo came out of retirement to work as a part-time security guard at the San Diego Convention Center during the Republican National Convention (1996). In 2003 he became a full-time security guard to help his youngest daughter purchase a home.

Donaldo lives in Chula Vista, California, with his wife. They lost one son and have three adult children, two grandchildren, and two great-grandchildren. He has written and published two other books, titled *Battling the Federal Gods* and *Warning: City Coffers Are Hungry*. Pending releases include three more books based on his life experiences: *Recovering a Stolen Vehicle from Mexico*, *In Search of a Thief*, and *The Adventures of a Security Guard*, as well as a book of short stories. He is a recognized local author with the San Diego Public Library.

www.ingramcontent.com/pod-product-compliance
Lightning Source LLC
Chambersburg PA
CBHW070005300526
45794CB00001B/190